SUN'S SEASON OF CHANNELS

SUN'S SEASON
OF CHANNELS

An Introduction to Chinese Philosophy,
Chinese Medical Theory and Channels

JONATHAN SHUBS

Illustrated by Fergus Byrne
Foreword by Simon Becker

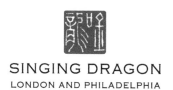

SINGING DRAGON
LONDON AND PHILADELPHIA

First published in Great Britain in 2021 by Singing Dragon,
an imprint of Jessica Kingsley Publishers
An Hachette Company

2

A CIP catalogue record for this title is available from the
British Library and the Library of Congress

ISBN 978 1 78775 902 2
eISBN 978 1 78775 903 9

Printed and bound in the United States by Integrated Books International

Jessica Kingsley Publishers' policy is to use papers that are natural, renewable and recyclable
products and made from wood grown in sustainable forests. The logging and manufacturing
processes are expected to conform to the environmental regulations of the country of origin.

Jessica Kingsley Publishers
Carmelite House
50 Victoria Embankment
London EC4Y 0DZ

www.singingdragon.com

Contents

Part III: The View of the Human Body in Channel Theory

Part IV: Understanding of the Channels

Part V: The Channels on the Body

Foreword

Stories make up the backbone of our lives. We communicate with stories. We think in stories, we experience in stories and we learn through stories. We remember stories that were told to us or that we were part of for many, many years. Stories shape how we think and who we are.

This also pertains to us as practitioners of Chinese medicine. Stories told to us about difficult cases, about clinical success, about personal experiences shape our understanding of this medicine.

Personally, stories told to me by Chinese medicine friends from around the world have hugely influenced my understanding and practice of our medicine. While I was a Chinese medicine student over 25 years ago in Florida, a senior student told me a story about the eclectic needle setting of the school director Dr. Su Liang Ku. To this day, this story influences how I needle my patients.

From a teacher's point of view, it is always easier to tell a story or a case history to illustrate a difficult point than to simply list theoretical facts. Also, I observe regularly how students studying herbs create elaborate stories around the name or look of a particular herb to help them memorize the functions. Even though the stories are much longer and certainly more complicated than the herb's functions, they are easier to remember than the two or three functions with their indications.

Likewise, some of the most important knowledge sources are case histories – stories about patients that are filled with rich information making the theory come alive. Prior to Chinese medicine being taught in university courses in the 1950s, this form of medicine was transmitted in a master disciple form in clinic where stories and particularly case histories dominated the form of teaching.

Clearly, stories are a key element in knowledge transmission. However, the entire first generation of Chinese medicine practitioners in the West has been educated with theory-laden textbooks that are filled with facts to be memorized. At the moment, there is a dire lack of didactic books for teaching Chinese medicine. Jonathan Shubs' *Sun's Season of Channels* begins to fill this void. It is one of the first books written specifically for students to learn the theory not by rote memorization but rather by way of a story, besides case history collections for more advanced practitioners.

Jonathan Shubs is a gifted teacher. After his lectures to our first-year students, I always meet many happy students in the hallway, telling me that Jonathan has been able to make the complicated material they have been struggling with accessible and clear. He does so by telling the stories that he now has laid out in this book. His teaching experience has shaped how he narrates his story.

Understanding the channel system is key in understanding acupuncture; however, many students struggle with this system for years. *Sun's Season of Channels* is a book for every student wanting to grasp the inherent logic of the intricate channel system in an easy and accessible way – in form of a story. Even more, this book is an entertaining read for practitioners wishing to a get a fresh perspective on the channel system.

Simon Becker, MSc, Director Chiway Academy

ACKNOWLEDGEMENTS

This book has been the work of many years. From the first concept to the various versions there were many people who helped me along the way.

First of all, I would like to thank all my students. Without their questions, comments, and desire to learn, this approach to understanding the channel system would not exist.

I would also like to thank my colleague Bijan Doroudian, who has worked with me on all the aspects of my teaching. I could not have written this book without his encouragement nor his feedback.

I would like to thank all the people who read the book in its various stages: Dave Shipsey, Anthony Monteith, Simon Becker, and Shana Shubs. Also my good friend Hiba Samawi, who read all the very early drafts and gave me constant encouragement throughout the whole writing process.

This book comes to life as a result of the wonderful illustrations of Fergus Byrne.

Finally, I would like to thank my two kids, Xavier and Adrien, for their constant questioning of everything. Their inquiring minds have been a major source of inspiration to me. I would also like to thank their mother, Elise Shubs, who has been a major support throughout my entire career.

INTRODUCTION

This book was conceived after teaching many students the channel or meridian system. Early in my career I was given the task of teaching channels to massage therapists, who did not know any Chinese medicine or channel theory, in five hours. This forced me to break down the whole system into its basic components and present them in a way that could be understood simply. The way I was taught the channels was the same as how most acupuncturists were taught, that is, to memorize the pathways with no explanation. It was purely a memorization approach that took many hours of study and revision. Having been a teacher of languages for many years, when I was confronted with this task of sharing the channels, I knew that a new approach was needed.

This book is the accumulation of years of working with hundreds of students and teaching them to understand the channels in a way that does not need memorization. My goal is to make the channel system accessible to everyone with no need for hours of study. This book will help new students of Chinese medicine prepare for learning about the channels, as well as any student of a healing modality that uses channels. This book is also aimed at anyone who has an interest in channels and Chinese medical philosophy.

The book is written as a dialogue. The two main classics of Chinese medicine (the *Huang Di Nei Jing* or *Sun Emperor's Classic of Chinese Medicine*, and the *Nan Jing* or *The Classic of Difficult Issues*) are both written as a discussion between the Yellow Emperor and his physician Qi Bo. The Yellow Emperor was a mythical emperor of China who was supposed to be highly cultivated and was the "perfect" emperor, and Qi Bo was the wise physician who was teaching his emperor and answering his questions. I took a similar approach to this book. I decided to make it a dialogue between a child named Sun and their grandparents, Grandmother and Grandfather Terra. This format is used for several reasons. First, it allows for the information to be presented in a storylike approach which helps make it more accessible. Second, it will prepare the student of Chinese medicine for this dialogue approach and it will feel familiar to seasoned practitioners. Last, it helps facilitate a learning process that is easier to retain. We remember stories more than we remember facts.

Each chapter is a conversation between Sun and Grandmother and Grandfather Terra. The chapters are ordered in a way that builds on the previous discussion and builds a full picture of the system. It is suggested that you read the book in order the first time. It can then serve as a quick reference for both theory and application of the channels.

A note on terminology

The word *meridian* has been used often to represent the system we are talking about in this book. In recent years, this term has been replaced by *channel*, as *channel* better represents a system of communication than *meridian*. I have chosen to use the word *channel* throughout the text to help reinforce this idea.

A note on pronouns and genders

The classics are written in a patriarchal way where only men could talk about important issues. To make this book more in line with my beliefs I have created a child called Sun who is neither a boy nor a girl. Sun is simply a child and will use the pronoun *they*.

1

SUN VISITS THEIR GRANDPARENTS

The low hum of the train was sending Sun to sleep. They were almost there. This was the moment they had been waiting for since last summer. They were finally going to be able to ask their questions and get the answers they so much wanted to know. But it was not just anticipation of understanding that had Sun excited. It was also that they were going to see their grandparents, and that they were on summer vacation. It had been a difficult year at school. Sun's teachers were happy with their progress, yet Sun felt that they were studying things that were not real. They wanted to understand the meaning of life and being, and this was not what they learned at school. This was the other reason Sun was excited—their grandparents. They were wise and talked to Sun like their equal, they always took their time to listen, and they did not tell Sun what to think but journeyed with them on their thoughts.

This summer was to be the big one. Sun's grandparents had given Sun books to read over the year, and now Sun was ready to discuss with them what they had read and understood. Sun's grandparents were both Chinese medicine doctors and were now retired, but still would travel the world to teach and inspire new acupuncturists. Sun loved their parents, but their grandparents were people they could relate to.

The train came to a slow stop in the station and Sun looked out the window. They saw their grandparents on the platform waiting for them. They looked just as solid and peaceful as ever. Sun started to feel at home just from seeing them.

After all the necessary formalities of greetings had been done, and as they were walking up the path to their small house in the countryside, Sun smiled to themselves. They felt at home.

Grandmother Terra led Sun up to Sun's room while Grandfather Terra went to the kitchen to start preparing tea. That was the tradition: every day at 4 p.m. they would sit on the porch overlooking the beautiful countryside and discuss. And today would be the first session.

"We will see you downstairs in ten minutes for tea," said Grandmother Terra as they left Sun to unpack.

2

THE DIFFICULTY OF GRASPING THE CLASSICS

Grandfather Terra brought the tea on to the back porch, poured a cup for his grandchild, wife, and himself, and then sat down in his favorite chair. He looked lovingly at his grandchild and asked, "How did you get on with the books we gave you at the end of last summer?"

Sun took a long sip of their tea, enjoying the flavor touching all the parts of their mouth, and then swallowed. They looked up at their grandfather, centered their thinking, and responded. "I read the classics that you gave me, the *Nei Jing* and the *Nan Jing*. There were times when I was confused, frustrated, and annoyed while reading these texts. And at other times I was thrilled, elated, and engaged. But overall, I feel like they are describing a world that can only be grasped at through words. There are times where I feel like they are hiding what they really want to say. Like they are being restrained from giving all the information. I also found it strange that many passages focused on geography or references that could only be Chinese. This is talking about a universal medicine that works on everyone, and yet these state that the human body is an image of China. I found this a bit difficult to come to terms with."

The two grandparents were beaming.

With a big smile, Grandfather Terra took in a breath and responded. "You have read with an open and still mind. You have read the classics well. They do give glimpses into the immensity of Chinese medicine and they are also opaque and difficult. This is for many reasons. First, they are written in an ancient language which is not used anymore. Ancient Chinese was a language of context and subtlety. The same character can be used in many different ways and can mean many different things. This is mainly based on context. The languages we read the classics in today are not the same language they were written in. So much of the nuance and subtlety is lost. Even those of us who read modern Mandarin have this problem. It is now a scholarly endeavor to read the classics in their original form.

"In addition to the language posing a barrier, there is also time and space. These books were written in a particular period in Chinese history. The original books were written in the Warring States period from around 700 to 300 BCE. This was a time of much political and social upheaval. Along with the classics of Chinese medicine we also find the development of the many philosophical schools during this period, the School of Yin and Yang, as well as that of the five elements or movements. And also, the great Taoist philosophers like Lao Tzu and Chuang Tzu lived during this time. And perhaps most importantly to the conception of the classics, Confucius lived during this time. China was a feudal society without an emperor. This lack of central power allowed for unprecedented free thought. This period is often compared to the Italian renaissance as the period of enlightenment.

"At the end of this period an emperor was able to unify all of China, and proceeded in burning all the writings that did not conform to his vision of society. From 213 to 206 BCE Terran Shi Huang systematically destroyed the literary history of China. The books we have today were rewritten after that period under the supervision of the emperor, which allowed him to control the way the intellectuals thought of him. As you read in the classics, often the body is compared to a well-run country, and the emperor is the most important organ. This is an example of the propaganda that was used to reinforce the importance of the emperor in everyday life.

"The medical scholars who rewrote the classics were only allowed to do so under the supervision of the emperor. They had to conform to the wishes and beliefs that were favored in the court at the time of writing. This was usually a Confucian ideology that promoted social cohesion and accepting one's place in society. With this weight of censorship, the scholars had to find ways of hinting at what the medicine behind the words was, but they had to be careful."

Sun had a look of intense thought, and then said, "I found it strange that the classics that I read did not talk about the history of how the system was discovered and developed. It was like this system of channels and Chinese medicine was sent from heaven and there was no process of understanding. But now that you have explained the historical and political context of these books, I see that they are just a glimpse at what was the real history of Chinese medicine. I felt that something was not quite right but now I get it. But this leads to another question. Why did you give me books to read if they are not the originals, have been manipulated for political ends, and are written in an ancient language that is difficult to decipher?"

Grandfather Terra replied, "It is important to know all these things. And yet there is still great wisdom and knowledge in these books. When you are aware of how, when, and why something is written you can put it into context. The writers still wanted to share the secrets of this healing modality. You just have to scrape the surface to get there. We will have much time to discuss this over the coming weeks, Sun. Now it is time to relax before dinner. We can continue tomorrow."

PART I

THE THEORY OF YIN AND YANG

3

THE ESSENCE OF
YIN AND YANG

Sun was impatient the next day. They were anxious to ask the plethora of questions that were running through their mind. And yet they knew that their grandparents would talk about the really important things only over tea. So, Sun had to bide their time until then.

Sun asked, "All the books I have read talk about Yin and Yang. I have gathered that they are two opposing and yet complementary forces. They are the basis of life and death and responsible for all the changes that we experience. They don't seem to be fixed references but rather dynamic forces that are in constant flux. Could you please enlighten me on this?"

Grandmother Terra looked at her grandchild with loving and compassionate eyes. A smile sneaked into the corners of her mouth as she closed her eyes to respond to the depth of Sun's question.

"You have grasped the essence of Yin and Yang. They are the cosmic interplay of opposing forces. They encompass everything that exists and are a modality to understand the world as a dynamic place that is in constant flux. This is the underlying message of the classics.

"Our medicine is to help the body be in harmony with its environment. When the interior and exterior are harmonious, so is our good health and wellbeing. To obtain this harmony we must first understand our place in our environment. As we mentioned before, the theory of channels was developed in ancient China, which was an agricultural society. The most important influence for any farmer is the cycle of the sun. When we closely observe all of nature, everything is based on the cycle of the sun. Day becoming night and the changes of the seasons are all expressions of the sun's cycles. When we talk about Yin and Yang, we are in essence talking about this cycle. The parts of the cycle in which the sun is more present are called Yang, and the absence of sun is called Yin. That which can be associated with the presence of the sun is more Yang, and that which is associated with the absence of the sun is more Yin.

"Now, as you mentioned, this is not a fixed association process but a dynamic flux. That which was Yin can become Yang, and that which was Yang can become Yin. Also, Yin cannot exist without Yang, and Yang cannot exist without Yin. Yin and Yang are opposing qualities that only exist when the other is present. In our language, it is like a comparative. To use the word 'hotter' I need two temperatures to compare. I cannot say Spain is hotter. I need to say Spain is hotter than another place for the sentence to make sense. This is true for Yin and Yang; I need to put Yang in contrast to Yin otherwise I am not talking about Yin and Yang."

Sun got excited; something clicked. "Grandmother Terra, I think I now grasp why they are said to be dynamic. If I use the example of 'hotter': Spain is hotter than Scotland, and at the same time Morocco is hotter than Spain. So, in this example, the relationship between Spain and Scotland, Spain would be more Yang, and in relation to Morocco it would be more Yin. Everything is in relation to something else.

Therefore, the characterization of Yin and Yang is relative to what is being talked about."

Grandmother Terra beamed with pride. "You have grasped the essence of Yin and Yang. Well done."

4

Yin and Yang and the Four Seasons

Sun asked, "Yin and Yang are two forces that only exist in context of each other. This I understand. Yet the seasons are said to be representations of Yin and Yang, and there are four seasons. How can Yin and Yang represent the four seasons when it is a relationship of two things?"

Grandfather Terra took a sip of tea and closed his eyes. After a moment he opened them and looked at Sun. He gathered his thoughts and then said, "Your observation is well founded. While Yin and Yang are two sides of the same coin and are binary, there is still room for subtlety. To do this we use layers. That is to say that we can look at Yin and Yang on different levels. Before we look at the seasons, let's look at a full night-and-day cycle. This cycle describes the arrival and disappearance of the sun in a 24-hour period. We can say that when there is sun the world is in a Yang phase, and when there is no sun the world is in a Yin phase. If we take, for example, March 21, we have 12 hours of Yang, when there is sunlight, and 12 hours of Yin, when there is no sun in the sky.

"We could leave it at that, and talk about day and night. Yet when we describe the cycle of the sun, we have morning, afternoon, evening, and night. These help us better understand where we are in the cycle of the sun, and to do this we need to add a second level of Yin and Yang.

"Now, the first representation of Yin and Yang was written in the *I Ching*, or the Book of Changes. In the *I Ching*, Yang is shown by a solid line and Yin by a broken line.

"So, just as Yin and Yang are two aspects of the whole, we can also say there will be two aspects of Yang and two aspects of Yin.

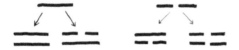

"And we can say that one aspect of the Yang base will be a Yang aspect and one will be Yin. And the same with the Yin base, one aspect being Yang and one being Yin.

"Let us call the bottom line the nature, or base, and the top line the change, or influence. So, regarding the Yang base, we have a Yang influence and a Yin influence. And likewise, regarding the Yin base we have a Yang influence and a Yin influence. We can also say that we have Yang within Yang and Yin within Yang on the Yang side, and Yang within Yin and Yin within Yin on the Yin side."

Sun remarked, "Here we have two aspects of Yin and two aspects of Yang. The two aspects of Yin are one being

Yin and the other being Yang, and the same is true for the Yang aspects. I think I get this. So, although we said that the presence of sun is Yang and the absence of sun is Yin, within the part of the day-night cycle that is day, there will also be a part which is Yin. And during the part of the cycle where there is absence of sun, there will be some Yang."

"Yes," smiled Grandmother Terra. "That is the gist of it. Now, how do we name the different aspects of the day and night cycle? We take that moment which has the most amount of sun, when the least amount of shadow is present, and call that Yang in Yang. In our language we would say midday, or 12 p.m. Logically we would place the Yin in Yin at the exact opposite time where there is the most shadow, which would be 12 a.m. or midnight.

"Now as you notice, after 12 p.m. the sun starts to set. Therefore, our strong base of Yang (sunlight) starts to slowly reduce. Or we could say that the shadows get bigger. Here we are having the presence of Yin influencing the Yang. So, we will say that dusk, or 6 p.m., is Yin in Yang. And the opposite would be true for dawn. The extreme Yin is starting to be influenced by Yang. The night which is maximum shadow starts to have the presence of light. Thus, dawn is Yang in Yin.

"So, we now have a cycle of the presence of the sun in relation to a 24-day cycle, and it looks like this:

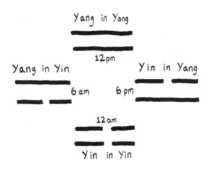

"So, we have two levels of Yin and Yang, the bottom being the main aspect and the top being the influence.

"Now, your question was about the seasons. And the seasons are another cycle of the sun, this time over a year instead of a day. So how do you think we would translate the same logic to the seasons?"

Sun picked up the pen and drew.

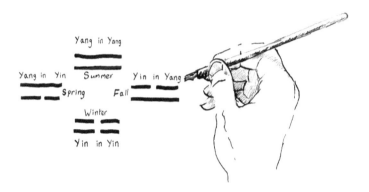

All three looked at each other, smiling. Sun explained their drawing. "As summer has the most sun, that would be Yang in Yang, and as winter has the least amount of sun, that would be Yin in Yin. Now, fall is when we have a good amount of sun, but it is diminishing. The foundation is Yang, but Yin is coming to change it and it would be Yin in Yang. Spring is the opposite of fall; we are coming out of the least sun and start to have the influence of the sun. Therefore, spring is Yang, the change, in Yin, the base."

All three were sipping their tea happily. Sun was finally understanding what they had only been grasping at before, and the grandparents were delighted that Sun was getting it.

"That is enough for one day," said Grandfather Terra. "Let us play some music before dinner."

PART II

THE THEORY OF
FIVE ELEMENTS

5

FOUR BECOMES FIVE

The next day went by very quickly. Sun did not notice the time pass. They were caught up in all that had been discussed the previous day and were getting their thoughts and questions ready for tea.

After a short nap in the afternoon Grandmother Terra called Sun to the back porch as Grandfather Terra was bringing out the tea.

"So," said Grandfather Terra as he was pouring the tea, "how have you been getting on today with our discussion yesterday?"

Sun responded, "I think I have understood the layers of Yin and Yang and how they relate to the cycle of the day/ night and the seasons. Yet, there is still one thing that is not very clear. In the classics it is mentioned that there are five seasons, not four. The balance and symmetry that the four variations of Yin and Yang have is almost perfect. It seems that adding a fifth element or position would break this. So, I guess my question is, how does four become five?"

"You don't miss a thing," Grandmother Terra responded. "That is the next problem to understand. And to understand it we have to go back to the beginning—the beginning of what there was before Yin and Yang. Where do Yin and Yang come from? As they are two sides of the same coin, what is the coin?"

Sun answered, "Before Yin and Yang everything was in an unformed state. If Yin and Yang are different perspectives of the same thing, then before, there was just the thing but no separation. All that Yin and Yang describe couldn't be described, because there was no contrast. It is like in science class when we are asked to describe what was before the Big Bang. It is impossible to describe it because we cannot compare it to anything. Or the only thing we can compare it to is what happened after the Big Bang. So we have separation of things now, but before we didn't."

"Brilliant," exclaimed Grandmother Terra. "Now we are getting somewhere. Let's look at the structure of what you have just said. The separation that we call Yin and Yang both come from the same source. This is also true for heaven and earth, heaven being Yang and earth being Yin. As they both come from the same point of origin, we call this point One. So we say One became Two. The One then broke into thousands of pieces and each of these pieces can be described from a point of view as being Yin or from another point of view as being Yang. The Big Bang is useful to understand the epicenter of this separation. When the separation happened, it started in a point and moved outward in all directions. There is a center, and all the pieces of the universe are around the center. Yin and Yang are describing the perspective from which we are witnessing this phenomenon. Yang is looking from the center, so we see the "light" reflected on things, and Yin is looking from the exterior, seeing things block the "light." So, in fact, Yin and Yang are perspectives of the One, and we can extrapolate that when we put Yin and Yang together, we are talking about the One: the universe from the two different vantage points together."

Sun was perplexed. They were sure they had grasped

everything yesterday and yet today it seemed more complicated. And then there was some clarity. "Everything starts in the center and the center is everything. The center explodes and all the fragments of everything start to move outward, away from the center. This movement creates two vantage points, looking toward the center and looking away from the center. Standing at the center looking out, you will see the center being reflected back at you, so this is Yang. Standing outside looking in, you will see the center being blocked by the forms of what is moving out from the center, and this is Yin. In essence, Yin and Yang are the same thing from two different perspectives and when together can describe all that is."

Grandfather Terra smiled. "Very well said, and now let's return to your original question. How does four become five? Do you remember how we got to four yesterday?"

"Of course," replied Sun as they took out the drawing from the previous discussion.

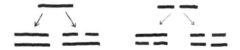

"Good," replied Grandfather Terra. "Now, notice that this is a top-down sequential diagram. By that, I mean the bottom group are derivatives of the top group. This is useful for progression of an idea, but it is not really representative of the universe. And it is important to remember that when we are talking about Chinese philosophy and medicine, we are trying to understand how the universe and then a person interacts with its environment. To do this we need a different setup that is more representative of the ebb and flow of things. We have already seen the second level, where there are two lines for each aspect, in a different alignment. Do you remember?"

Again, Sun took out the diagram and showed it to their grandfather.

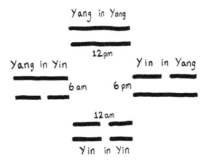

"And now if we take out all the words and just have a diagram?"

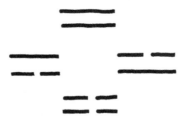

"Good; and now where do you think the first level will go from the sequential diagram?"

Sun knew right away, and drew it in the center.

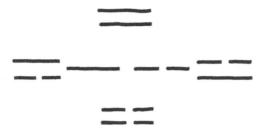

Grandmother Terra explained, "We have the four aspects of Yin and Yang forming a circle and the original separation of Yin and Yang in the center creating the fifth place. So, now we have five out of four. And how do we place the seasons around this?"

Sun thought and then spoke. "Well, I don't imagine that the placement of the seasons from yesterday will change, so I can only imagine that the middle, or the center, will be the fifth season. However, if we separate the cycle of the earth around the sun into five sections or seasons, I don't see where the fifth season would go. Anywhere it gets put will sort of destroy the ebb and flow of the other seasons."

Grandmother Terra replied, "You are partly correct. If we leave it as a whole section of the cycle, then it would not be well balanced. And unfortunately, this is how the five seasons have been misinterpreted in the West for some time. In many books they placed the fifth season as late summer. And when we are asked about this in our courses, we respond that late summer is a quarter correct. Let me explain.

"Let's take a step back first and just put some ideas on the table. We have said that there are five seasons, and we have 365 days in a year. How many days will each season be?"

"Three hundred and sixty-five divided by five is 73, so there will be 73 days in a season. But I still don't see where the fifth season goes?"

"Patience, we will get there. So, we will have 73 days of summer (Yang in Yang), 73 days of winter (Yin in Yin), 73 days of spring (Yang in Yin), and 73 days of fall (Yin in Yang). That leaves us with 73 days of this fifth season. After the 73 days of summer, do you think we go directly to the 73 days of fall?"

"Well, there would be a transition, I guess, like a buffer. I don't feel that it is summer one day and fall the next. It is gradual. So…the period between the seasons would be the fifth season. And as there are four transitions there would be four segments of the fifth season. And this would mean that the fifth season would not be continuous, but it would be separated by the other seasons."

"And how long would each of those four segments of the transition season last for?"

"Well, 73 divided by 4 is 18.25; 18 days, I would guess."

Grandfather Terra chuckled. "We can see math is going well for you at school. Yes, so to recap, we have five seasons. The four seasons we are used to each last for 73 days, and we have a transition period of 18 days between each season. Now I have a question for you, Sun. When is the first day of spring?"

Sun replied, "March 21 of course. Everyone knows that."

Grandfather Terra smiled. "In the West, yes, you are correct. We say that spring starts on the day of the spring equinox. And if we were to look at it from a Chinese point of view, where the equinox is the perfect balance of day and night, does that describe the beginning of a period or the middle? If we think about it as a wave, we will see the seasons as such.

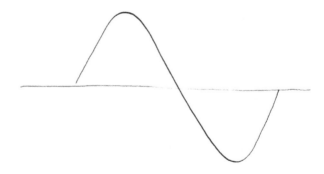

"And then we say that Yang in Yang is the very top of the wave.

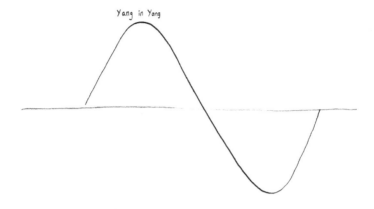

"We would not say that Yang in Yang *starts* at the top, but that it is *at its zenith* at the top. There will be a part of Yang in Yang before the zenith and a part after the zenith. So, we would have something like the following.

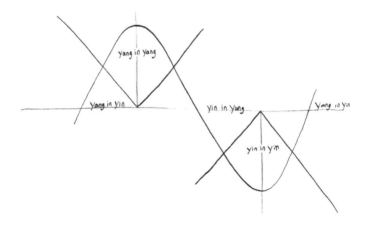

"We can see that each of the four aspects occupy different spaces along the wave. And their pure sense is directly in the middle of the area they occupy in the wave. If we are then to put this on the seasons, we would have a wave that looks like this.

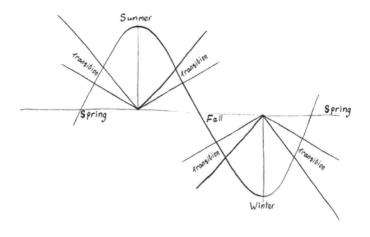

"So, now when would you think spring starts?"

Sun thought and looked at the pictures and finally said, "The spring equinox is the middle of the season, the season is one-fifth of a year, which is 73 days, and as the equinox is the middle we need to go 36 days before March 21." And then they took out a piece of paper and drew.

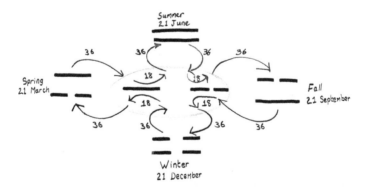

Grandfather Terra exclaimed, "Yes, that is exactly correct. We see 36 days before and after each equinox and solstice to define the whole period of the season, and four cycles of

18 days between each season. So, if we were to write out the dates, we would get something like this."

```
Spring                                    5 February - 17 April
Transition from Spring to Summer  ——  18 April - 4 May
Summer                             ——   5 May - 17 July
Transition from Summer to Fall     ——  18 July - 4 August
Fall                               ——   5 August - 17 October
Transition from Fall to Winter     ——  18 October - 4 November
Winter                             ——   5 November - 17 January
Transition from Winter to Spring   ——  18 January - 4 February
```

Sun said, "The seasons in Chinese thought are not based on the climatic changes that differ from one place to another. They are based on the quantity of sun that the place gets. And it would follow that if we were in the southern hemisphere then the dates would be inversed. But the cycle would still be the same. This model will work anywhere on earth.

"I see now how four becomes five."

Both grandparents were happy with Sun. They had made some great leaps of logic and understood. And they were all tired. Grandmother Terra started to clear up the tea as Grandfather Terra started to put away the drawings they had made. They both saw the slight look of disappointment on Sun's face.

"That is enough for one day, Sun. You have a lot to digest and we haven't even eaten dinner yet."

Sun smiled and knew that was all for today.

6

FROM SEASONS TO ELEMENTS

Sun came down the stairs ready for breakfast feeling slightly overwhelmed and at the same time excited by the previous day's discussion. They were anxious to start the day and even more to get to teatime, but they would have to wait, for that wasn't for another few hours.

They walked into the kitchen to see both grandparents bustling about more than usual. Not only was breakfast ready, there were backpacks lying by the door.

"What's going on?" asked Sun.

"We are going on a hike today," answered Grandmother Terra. "Have your breakfast and then go get ready."

"Will we be back for teatime?" asked Sun.

Grandfather Terra chuckled. "Go get ready and don't worry—we will have our time to talk."

They left the house shortly after breakfast, each of them with a backpack and walking stick ready for the day's adventure. Unlike their normal hikes around the lake, this time they headed off toward the mountain where the old mine was. They followed the river to the base of the mountain and then started to walk by the stream. The woods were all around them and the smell of the leaves was intoxicating. Sun was taking all this in when their grandparents stopped at a clearing and declared, "Time to stop and make lunch."

While Grandmother Terra made a small fire, Sun went to get some water from the stream. By the time they came back the fire was going and the smell of roasting fish that Grandfather Terra had caught that morning helped Sun realize how hungry they actually were.

After a good meal of fish and bread, the grandparents started to boil water for some tea.

"If you are making tea then we get to talk," exclaimed Sun.

"Darn right," replied Grandmother Terra. "And this is the perfect place to do it."

Without missing a moment Sun dived right in. "We talked about how there are five different seasons and how they are reflections of the amount of sunlight that the earth gets during that period. The number five is used in the classics in reference to the elements. How do the seasons relate to the elements, and how do the elements relate to each other?"

With a grin, Grandmother Terra replied, "That was the question we were hoping you would ask, and that is the reason for our hike. The idea of the five elements, or the five movements as they are sometimes referred to, is the second cornerstone of Chinese thought after Yin and Yang. Just like with the seasons, the elements are an attempt to understand the world around us and how all the different components interact. The Chinese identified five different elements or phenomena that were necessary for their lives. To begin with they looked at what they as humans needed for their basic functions—food and water. Looking at all the food sources, they realized that all food came from plants in some way. So, the first element was plant, or *wood*. And to complement the wood they needed *water*. Next, they looked at their comfort, and for this they needed heat, which came from *fire*. Next, they needed tools, and these were made from *metal*. Finally, all four phenomena were taken or produced in some way from the earth. So, the five elements were:

Wood

Water

Fire

Metal

Earth.

"And each of these elements could be related to a season.

"The seasons were associated with the elements based on what was happening in that season.

"In spring, plant life starts, and trees start to come back to life, so wood is associated with spring.

"In summer, the earth gets scorched and there are forest fires, so summer is associated with fire.

"In fall, the harvest is happening, and to do this we need tools to cut the grain, so fall is associated with metal.

"In winter, things are cold and the coldest element is water, so winter is associated with water.

"And in the interseason, there is transition, and earth is the transition for all the other elements, so interseason is associated with earth."

"OK, that makes sense," said Sun. "Would that also mean that the different levels of Yin and Yang that we associate with the seasons could also be associated with the elements?"

"Yes," replied Grandfather Terra. "The pictures we made yesterday can be adapted as such."

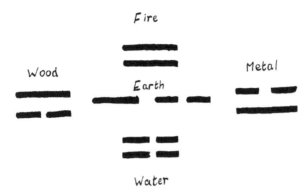

7

THE ASSOCIATIONS OF
THE FIVE ELEMENTS

"We started with Yin and Yang," said Sun. "If something is Yin then it is compared to another thing that is Yang. This is simple because there are two things being compared to each other. Now we have five elements. It seems much more complicated to compare one thing to four other things. As there are more categories there must be more subtleties in how they are compared. This seems quite difficult."

"Good observation," replied Grandfather Terra. "The five elements are slightly different in the way that we associate different things to them. It is true that each represents a dynamic of Yin and Yang, as do the seasons. When we take different categories, we then break the category down into five aspects. Each of these aspects is an element. So, within a group of five things, we can associate each thing with one element. We already did this with the seasons. Let's do it with climatic factors. So, there are five main climatic factors, wind, heat, dampness, dryness, and cold. Each of these can be associated with an element. How would you associate them?"

Sun thought for a moment, then said, "Three are easy and two are more difficult. Heat I would associate with fire as fire makes heat. Water is with cold, as the coldest thing I can think of is ice, which is water. The trees and wind are closely related, so I would associate wind with wood. Now it gets a bit tricky. I have dryness and dampness left, and earth and metal. Perhaps I would associate dampness with earth, as earth is often moist and I remember learning that basements that are underground can get lots of mildew which is caused by dampness. So, dampness is with earth, and that would leave dryness with metal. I don't really see the dryness-to-metal relationship except that it is the only one left."

"Yes, dryness with metal is a little more difficult. The best explanation I think is to look at what happens to metal when it gets wet or humid. It starts to rust. Metal does not like to be wet. This is one reason why it needs to be dry, and thus we associate dryness with metal. And this also shows that the associations are not always perfect. Whereas the associations of the other four elements are clear, metal is not so clear in this case. This is something that comes up often in studying the five elements. Some things are very clear, and some are a bit more difficult to understand. Would you like to try another association?"

Sun nodded.

"How about directions? There are the four directions and the center. How would you associate them with the five elements?"

Sun thought for a moment again and then answered. "I will use the movement of the sun and the levels of Yin and Yang that are associated with each element to help me. The sun rises in the east, and that is daybreak. We saw that daybreak was Yang over Yin and associated with wood. So wood is the east, and exactly opposite the east is the west. The opposite of Yang over Yin is Yin over Yang and that was sunset and metal. So east is wood, and west is metal. I would then think that the further north we go the colder it gets. Cold is with water as it is Yin in Yin, so water is north, and that would mean the south is fire. I would then imagine that the earth is the center."

"Very good," said Grandmother Terra. "In Chinese history the south was always put at the top of the page or map. There are many other categories that can be then associated with each of the elements. For example, colors:

Fire—red

Water—black

Metal—white

Wood—green

Earth—yellow.

"Or emotions:

Fire—joy

Water—fear

Metal—sadness

Wood—anger

Earth—overthinking.

"We could go on and on, but I think you have got the idea."

"OK, I get it," exclaimed Sun. "Yet to be honest, the idea of associations, although interesting, seems a little static. I mean, to categorize things can be fun and, in some ways, useful, I guess. But I'm struggling to see how this really helps to understand how nature works. It is like saying that night, winter, female, and so on are Yin. It lacks complexity."

Grandmother Terra let out a big laugh and looked at Grandfather Terra with a glint in her eye. Their exchange was full of admiration for Sun's quick thinking. Their grandchild was special indeed.

8

THE MOVEMENTS OF
THE FIVE ELEMENTS

Sun was not amused. Were their grandparents laughing at them? All they did was ask a simple question. "Why are you laughing? I was just observing that the five elements seemed static when used as a means to categorize different things. I don't think I said anything funny."

"Not at all, Sun," responded Grandmother Terra. "We were laughing because talking to you is an absolute pleasure. You know that your grandfather and I have been teaching for many years and we are amazed at how quickly you make the connections. Sharing our knowledge with you is a pleasure, and we were laughing in pure delight."

"OK. I guess that makes sense. I'll let it go." Sun was trying to hide the pride they felt while they talked. "So, are you going to tell me how the five elements become dynamic, or do I have to figure it out for myself?" There was a hint of mischief in their voice.

Grandfather Terra took his time pouring everyone a new cup of tea. He then sat down next to Sun and took out the pad of paper and a pen.

"You are correct in stating that the five elements as a

system to classify categories does seem static if we stop at that, just as Yin and Yang are static when they are only used to classify things. However, the five elements also have a dynamic aspect as well. To see this, we need to arrange the five elements slightly differently. When we use the image we've been using so far it doesn't give itself to showing interactivity. We have five different elements, and if we want them all to interact there has to be space for them to interact. So, instead of keeping them as top, bottom, left, right, and center, we will put them all around in a circle. Using the picture below, how will we do this?"

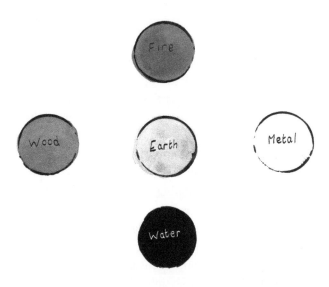

Sun responded, "Fire, metal, water, and wood are already at the perimeter of the picture. I would think the easiest thing to do is to put earth also at the exterior. However, I don't see where it would go. There is logic for putting it between any of the elements, as all the elements come from earth to begin with."

"Indeed. And the reason we place earth in a particular

place will become clearer once we see the circular system in action. So, for the time being, please let the questioning mind rest while we explain the system and then see if the questions still arise."

"OK. I will try to, but no promises," responded Sun, a bit cheekily.

"Thank you for trying," Grandfather Terra said with a laugh. "To stop you asking where it goes, I will now tell you. Earth is placed between fire and metal. This gives us the following picture." He quickly drew in his book, then showed Sun what he had drawn.

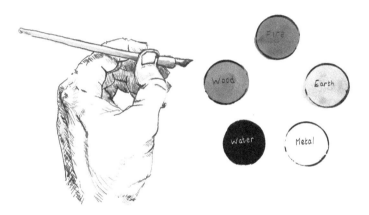

Grandmother Terra refilled the teacups and said, "When the elements are arranged in this way, we can now see how they interact. We will look at two types of interactions. When we talk about five elements, we call the interactions *cycles*, because they create a full cycle and touch each element in a specific pattern. The first of these cycles is called the generating cycle. In this cycle we move around the circle clockwise. And we say that each element generates or nourishes the element after it. Here we are in the forest surrounded by trees. These trees need one thing besides the sun to grow."

"Water, they need water. Everyone knows that," Sun said, not able to hold back.

"Yes, wood needs water to grow, so water nourishes wood. We just had lunch and made a fire to boil the water. When the fire was dying down, we added more wood to the fire to increase the heat. So…"

"So, wood nourishes fire. Got it."

"Perfect. Now, the teacups we are drinking out of are made from clay, which is earth. When they were formed, they were very weak and fragile. Once they were put in a kiln or oven, they became strong. So, fire nourishes and reinforces earth. Do you know what is at the top of this mountain?" Grandmother Terra pointed to the path that led up to the summit.

"There's an old gold mine. We visited it a few summers ago," responded Sun.

"Yes. The opening to the mine is halfway up this trail. That mine goes down very deep underground where the gold deposits are. It is deep in the ground or earth where metal comes together. Earth nourishes and helps metal to become greater. So, earth nourishes metal."

"Sun, where is the freshest and cleanest water?"

"Hmm, difficult to say. I would think a stream high in the mountains, one where there are lots of rocks around. That is always my favorite water," Sun responded, remembering drinking from the stream earlier.

"Exactly. It is the minerals that are in the rocks that purify and clean the water. So, metal, which includes minerals, nourishes water.

"As we have seen, water nourishes wood. We have come full circle. Each element nourishes the element after it in a clockwise rotation, and is nourished by the element before it. We call this the generating or nourishing cycle, and it looks like this." Grandmother Terra took the image of the elements in a circle and added five arrows.

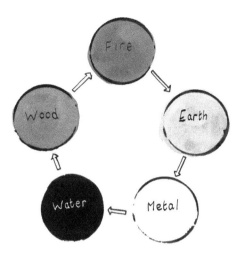

Sun looked at the image and said, "So each element is nourished by one element and nourishes another element. Wood nourishes fire and is nourished by water, fire nourishes earth and is nourished by wood, earth nourishes metal and is nourished by fire, metal nourishes water and is nourished by earth, and finally water nourishes wood and is nourished by metal. I get it.

"You said there were two cycles. If in this first cycle each element interacts with two elements, then in the second cycle would the element interact with the other two elements it doesn't interact with in this cycle?"

"You said you were going to calm your questioning mind," said Grandfather Terra with a laugh. "It is your nature, so we shouldn't be surprised. You are correct, Sun, the second cycle will complete all the interactions. The second cycle is called the controlling cycle. When we nourish something, it can grow. We also need a counterinfluence to help it grow in the correct way. If not, it will just not stop growing, and this can be a problem. So, each element will control or help structure another element when it is too strong.

"What will we do to the fire when we finish our talk here and leave the campsite?"

"Well, as you always taught me, we have to make sure the fire is out. So, we will put water over it."

"Exactly. When fire gets out of control, we pour water on it. So, water controls fire.

"Now, do you remember when we visited the blacksmith a few years back?"

"I do—when we went to see him make the iron rods for the porch."

"And how did he make it so he could form and manipulate the iron?"

"He heated it up and then banged it into shape. Let me guess—the fire made it so he could work with the metal, so fire controls metal."

"Nothing gets by you, Sun. Now think about the bamboo growing in our garden. What do we do when it gets too big?"

"We cut or chop it down."

"Exactly, and we use a metal blade to cut or chop it down. So, metal controls wood.

"We are sitting here in the forest. When we touch the soil, it is damp and stays in place. When you went to the desert with your parents last year do you remember the landscape?"

"It was barren. There were almost no trees and the sand was moving everywhere."

"Exactly. The trees and plants help the soil and earth to stay put. If a big gust of wind blows across the desert all the sand moves. When the same happens in the forest, the trees hold the earth in place, and it doesn't move around. Therefore, wood controls earth.

"Now look at the stream over there. There is water running down the hill. What is on either side of the water, and what contains the water, so it doesn't go everywhere?"

"The banks of the riverbed. And I can guess you will tell me that they are made of earth. And if I think of all bodies of water, they are all contained by earth. This is true for oceans, seas, lakes, rivers, and so on. And now we can say that earth controls water.

"I get it. The control cycle has a similar pattern to the generating cycle except that it is not interacting with the element next to it, but it jumps an element. So, water controls fire and is controlled by earth, fire controls metal and is controlled by water, metal controls wood and is controlled by fire, wood controls earth and is controlled by metal, and finally earth controls water and is controlled by wood."

Grandmother Terra took out the paper again and drew a new diagram.

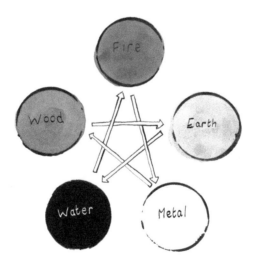

"When we put both cycles together, we get the following," said Grandmother Terra.

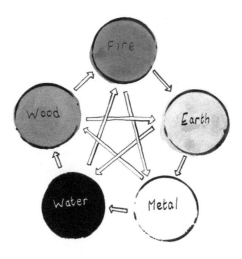

"And here we can see that each element interacts with each other element in either the nourishing or control cycle.

Fire nourishes earth, controls metal, gets controlled by water, and gets nourished by wood.

Earth nourishes metal, controls water, gets controlled by wood, and gets nourished by fire.

Metal nourishes water, controls wood, gets controlled by fire, and gets nourished by earth.

Water nourishes wood, controls fire, gets controlled by earth, and gets nourished by metal.

Wood nourishes fire, controls earth, gets controlled by metal, and gets nourished by water.

"This is how the five elements become dynamic. Every element interacts with each other through a different relationship. When one element changes it has an effect on each other element. They are all interdependent and interact with each other."

Sun saw it. "OK. I now see how the elements can be dynamic. And the reason that earth is placed between fire and metal is because of the nature of the relationships it has with the other elements. I just have one question left."

"Another question? Don't you ever stop?" said Grandfather Terra jokingly.

"Did you two plan this hike and this picnic on purpose to help explain the elements to me?"

They all laughed. Sun's grandparents glanced at each other and then nodded. They all knew that was the end of today's talk.

PART III

THE VIEW OF THE HUMAN BODY IN CHANNEL THEORY

9

Yin and Yang in Relationship to the Human Body

The previous day's hike had been a great success. Sun was very pleased with their new understanding of the five elements and enjoyed the nature walk. They were sure today would be just as informative, and were looking forward to teatime to see what was next. Sun went downstairs and had breakfast. They overheard their grandparents talking and stopped to hear what they were saying.

"Sun has really grasped everything so far. They are much quicker than I expected," said Grandmother Terra.

"Yes," replied Grandfather Terra. "They could easily join our university courses and not miss a thing. I'm a bit apprehensive though about the next step. We have finished the general ideas and are now going to have to start talking about how all this relates to the human body. This will get more complex, and I think we should take it more slowly."

"I know what you are thinking. I'm sure they will continue to surprise us, but perhaps you are correct. Let's ease into the applications of these ideas to the human body slowly. Once they start to get the main ideas, I am sure it will go well."

Sun walked into the room making enough noise to announce their arrival. "Good morning. Listen, I was thinking after yesterday's hike and talk. We have been talking a lot about big theories. We still haven't talked once about the human body and how all this relates to the channels. And I would like to remind you that we agreed this summer you would be teaching me about the channel system. So, if you both agree, perhaps we could start with that today? I already have many questions ready and many ideas that I would like to get more clarity on. Anyways, I'm sure you know best."

Sun was smiling inside. They were sure their grandparents now had no choice but to push ahead. Sun was going to take the initiative and start accelerating things. They decided that it was time to try to extend the conversations to beyond just teatime.

"Last night in bed I was trying to see how Yin and Yang and the five elements are related to the channels. I remember that in the classics some channels were classified as Yang and others Yin. Also, the channels have Chinese names and organs attached to them. I have a feeling that all this comes together somehow. Perhaps you could give me some slight insight, so my questions are more refined when we talk?"

Sun was counting on their grandparents' love of teaching overriding their rule of only talking over tea. They both loved sharing knowledge, and Sun knew they were trying to resist.

It was Grandmother Terra who gave in first. "You're correct Sun. They all tie together, and I guess it won't hurt to talk a little outside of teatime. It was, after all, us who gave the opening with the hike yesterday. All right—let's talk about Yin and Yang as they relate to the human body, and then save the other questions for later."

Sun was happy with this new development. "Yin and Yang are references to the sun. I would imagine that when we talk about Yin and Yang, we are referring to the amount of sun the body gets. But the body moves all the time and its relationship to the sun would change too. How, then, do we say which part of the body is Yang or Yin?"

"Always to the heart of it, eh?" responded Grandfather Terra. "You are correct. The body is always moving, and when we are talking about Yin and Yang they too are always moving. The answer to this is to take the body in its most common postures in regard to the sun and then classify the Yin and Yang based on these postures. What do I mean by this? Well, first we should remember that the channels are part of the healing system whose main modality is acupuncture. This modality was created over 3000 years ago in ancient China. China was at this time, and still is to this day, a mainly agricultural society. The majority of the population were farmers and worked in the fields. When people are working in the fields they are usually slightly bent forward. When a person is slightly bent forward the majority of the sunlight will land on their back. So, the back portion of the body is more Yang and the front portion of the body is more Yin."

Sun nodded and smiled. "I can see that the teacher has awakened in you, Grandfather. You can't help yourself."

Laughing at himself, Grandfather Terra responded, "Yes. When I start talking about the human body, I tend to go into teacher mode. We will try to keep it simple. As you stated, we use the sun to determine which parts of the body are labeled Yin or Yang. And as with everything else, it is always in relation to another part of the body. There are two main ways in which we look at the body when we talk about Yin and Yang. The first is on a vertical plane. Here we mean that, going from the head to the feet, we divide the body along the front and the back, and the interior and the exterior. The front and the interior get less sun so are Yin, and the back and exterior get more sun so are Yang."

"OK. My belly compared to my back would be Yin, and my back in relation to my belly is Yang. That is the front and back part. What do you mean by interior and exterior though?"

Grandmother Terra chimed in. "Stand up, Sun. Let your hands dangle at your sides. The part of your arm that is at the exterior is the part that is not touching your body, and the part that is the interior is the part touching your body. Look at your hand from the side. When you look at your hand with the thumb above and the pinky below, do you see a change in skin color along the thumb, one part white and the other part more colored?"

"Yes, I see that. The white part covers my palm and the colored part covers the back of my hand. So the white part is Yin and the colored part is Yang?"

"Exactly, and when you hold out your arm in front of you with the thumb up and the pinky down and follow those lines up the arm, they also show that the interior side or palm side is Yin and the back of the hand side is Yang."

"And the legs?" asked Sun.

"When you are standing up, imagine a line going vertically through the center of the knee cap. The interior side of that line is Yin and the exterior side is Yang."

Sun asked, "When I am standing up and the inner parts of my thighs are touching, that would be the center line of the Yin aspect of my leg, and the outer seam of my trousers would show the middle of the Yang side of my leg?"

"Exactly. The seams in your jeans are going along the middle of the Yin and Yang sides. So half in front of the seams and halfway behind the seams is where Yin and Yang meet on the leg."

"Got it. So, the arms and the legs are clear. When standing with my arms hanging by my sides the exterior parts of my arms and legs are Yang and the interior sides are Yin. How about the body and the head?"

Grandfather Terra responded, "The head is the highest part of the body and closest to the sun. The whole head is Yang. On the body the whole back is Yang, and the front of the body is Yin. Careful though, as there are some Yang channels on the front of the body. This, however, we will talk about when we look at the channels in more detail."

Sun said, "The exterior of the arms and legs are Yang along with the head and back. The interior of the arms and legs are Yin along with the front of the body. However, for the front there are some portions that are Yang and some that are Yin, and we will see that more when we get further into the channels. Great. Now, will you two please stop talking so I can eat my breakfast. Really."

They all laughed, and Sun was proud at having succeeded in getting their grandparents to talk.

10

WHAT EXACTLY IS A CHANNEL?

After a day of gardening and enjoying the balmy summer weather, Sun and their grandparents sat down for their afternoon tea. As usual, Grandfather Terra poured the tea and then they all settled in for their afternoon talk. Sun was still happy with their ruse to get their grandparents to talk that morning and didn't want to push it too much. Yet, there was one question they had been waiting to ask since breakfast time.

Sun started, "This morning we were talking about how Yin and Yang are applied to the human body. At the end you mentioned channels and that some channels were Yin, and some were Yang. When people talk about acupuncture and when I read the classic books these are mentioned too. And yet, I have not been able to grasp fully what a channel is. Could you help me better understand the meaning of channels?"

Grandfather Terra chuckled. "Yes, you did get us to talk this morning. You are a wily one indeed. Channels. What are they? This is an excellent question. When we are talking about channels, we are referring to the Chinese word *Jing*. The word has two meanings: first, of a place where things move within, like a channel, and second, a geographical meaning which is close to longitude. These two aspects together give us an idea of what is meant by *channel*. So, I guess we could say it is a vertical division of the body that things move in.

"To begin, the geographical aspect is easier to understand. Think of a globe, for example. If we want to pinpoint a position on the globe, we need to have two pieces of information, longitude and latitude. Longitudinal lines go from the North Pole to the South Pole, and latitudinal lines are horizontal circles that go around the globe from east to west. They are like Y versus X graphs where Y is the vertical axis and X the horizontal axis.

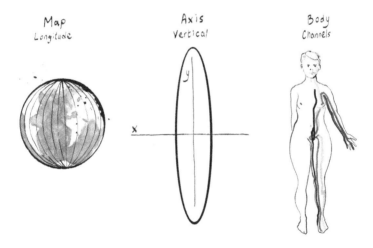

"So, we use the channels to give vertical segments that we can then use to identify where we are on the body. We can say that the Qi moves within these vertical segments. And depending on where the segment is on the body and the amount of sunlight it gets, it may have a different type of Qi. And before you ask, we will talk about what Qi is later."

"OK," said Sun. "So, the channels are these vertical portions of the body and Qi moves in them. What about the horizontal axis of the body? If channels are the vertical plane, what is the horizontal plane?"

Grandmother Terra responded, "Well, we use the bones and muscles. See, look at your left knee. You know exactly where to look. Now, *where* on your left knee should you look? That is where the channels come in. A channel on the left elbow is an exact place."

Sun started to look at their elbow and understood.

11

THE MYSTERIOUS QI

Sun was still thinking about the channels when a question came to mind.

"You said that channels were vertical segments of the body, and that was the geographical aspect of the word *Jing*. And you also said that Jing was a channel or conduit. And then you mentioned Qi, saying that Qi was in the channel. What is Qi?"

Grandmother Terra smiled. She had been waiting for this question. "Well. That is a big question. The word *Qi* has many meanings in Chinese medicine and its definition is hard to grasp. Even amongst acupuncturists and Chinese medicine practitioners there is much debate about this. I will try to give you an idea all the same.

"The ideogram of Qi is of steam rising from uncooked rice, and it is said that Qi is the energy that makes up everything. One interpretation is that Qi incorporates everything, from solid uncooked rice to the gas state of steam, meaning that it has all three forms of matter and can also be that which changes the matter. We could also look at it as the potential of everything and the manifestation of everything."

Grandmother Terra saw that Sun looked confused. She thought for a moment and then pointed at the cup in her hand. "You see this cup, Sun? We call it a cup because it has a form that we recognize, and the form also has a function that we recognize. The shape of the object is defined by its physical occupation of space. This is the manifested aspect of the cup and the manifested Qi of the cup.

"The physical aspect of the cup is also defined by the empty space where the cup is not. The hollow center that the cup defines gives the object a function. The empty space in the middle allows the cup to be used to hold liquid, which is its function. Without the empty space it would not be a cup and not have a function. So, Qi can refer to the form of the cup and the function of the cup. It is both the physical manifested form as well as the function and its potential."

Sun exhaled; they were trying to comprehend what their grandmother was saying. They understood in broad strokes, but it still felt like they were not quite getting it. They said, "I can see that it is a subtle idea to grasp. It seems like Qi is everything in the universe. And not just the physical matter—it is also all the changes and possible changes of the matter. And it seems to also be the interactions this matter has with other matter and the potential interactions with other matter. Is it a word that is used to describe all that is, was, and will be?"

Grandmother Terra smiled. "Yes. That is a good description of Qi. It is matter in all its forms, the function of the matter in all its functions, and the potential for those forms and functions to change. It is the vast universe and the smallest subatomic particles and everything in between. Basically, it is everything and all that everything can be."

Sun was nodding. They understood the vastness of it and the all-encompassing idea of Qi. When this understanding became more concrete in their mind, a new question arose. "Qi is everything that makes up our world, from the physical matter to the function of the matter and the possible changes of the matter and the function. This is a vast concept and all-encompassing. And yet in the classics they talk about how Qi flows in the channels and that there are different types of Qi. They say that each organ has a special type of Qi. What do they mean by this?"

Grandfather Terra was happy to respond to this question. "You are correct, Sun. The broad definition of Qi is a vast all-encompassing idea that includes all in the universe. When we talk about Qi in Chinese medicine and in the channels, we are mainly referring to the function and potential changes aspect of Qi. In the channels, we say that Qi flows. This means that in the channels there is the potential to change something in the body. This is very important for acupuncture. We insert needles into places on the body. Depending on the channel we place the needle in, we are stimulating a particular potential for change. We could say that the potential for change is what flows in the channels.

"When we talk about the different types of Qi we are talking about a function. If we say Lung Qi, we are talking about all the functions that are associated with the Lung organ in Chinese medicine. And if we talk about defensive Qi, we are referring to the function of defending the body. Often in Chinese medicine we can think of Qi as function or potential of change.

"When we are talking about the body, we can say that everything is Qi, from the physical forms—bones, flesh, organs, blood vessels, tissues, fluids, and so on—to the functions of the physical forms—breathing, digesting, pumping blood, and so on—to the emotional and spiritual forms. All of this in the pure sense is Qi.

"However, we have a more limited meaning when we also talk about Qi in relation to the human body. It is the function of change and movement—this we call Qi. When we talk about the ability to support or nourish something, we call this *blood*. And when we talk about the emotional, psychological, or spiritual aspect, we call this *spirit*. This gives us three different aspects of the great Qi. The most physical and nutritive aspect we call *blood*. The function of the body and its changes we call Qi. And finally, the most subtle changes of the connection to the universe we call *spirit*."

Sun was confused again and tried to put it together. "As you have told me, there are two main explanations of Qi: one in a general sense where it is everything in the universe, and a second which is specific to Chinese medicine, where it is the function and potential for change. This second use is what the classics are referring to. In this use it is a way of talking about the functions and potential for change and differentiating that aspect from the nutritive aspect and the spiritual aspect. If I were to use the ideas of Yin and Yang to describe these three things (blood, Qi, and spirit), I could say that as blood is the most nutritive and more supporting it would be more Yin. Spirit, which is the most subtle and abstract, would be most Yang. That would leave Qi being the function and potential for change in the middle. More Yang than blood, and more Yin than spirit."

Grandmother Terra exhaled and smiled. "Sun, it is a pleasure to share our knowledge with you. You get it. And we are proud of you…"

Grandfather Terra interrupted. "Sun, everything your grandmother said is true. And please don't let that go to your head. But you can let our love go to your heart."

They all knew that the tea was cold, and it was time for dinner.

12

THE INTERNAL ORGANS AND THE BOWELS

The morning after the discussion about Qi, Sun's mind was swimming in the knowledge and struggling to keep their head above water. Everywhere they looked they saw Qi. They started thinking about every object's form, function, and potential for change. They were captivated by how simple a concept it was and yet how all-engulfing it was. They were lost in their thoughts while doing all the household activities of the day. They had to replant the same flower five times before they got it right. When it was teatime, they were full of wonder at the universe.

The tea service was ready on the porch, and Grandfather Terra was already pouring the tea when Sun arrived. He poured Sun a cup and looked up with a smile. "You have been silent today, Sun. What is going on in your mind?"

"I've been thinking about Qi. How it is everywhere and is everything. About its relationship to the channels and the human body. And when I think about it, new questions come into my mind."

Grandmother Terra said warmly, "Of course it opens new

questions. That is the result of getting answers. Where has your mind been taking you today?"

"I've been thinking about functions—functions in the human body. When I was planting the new roses in the garden, I saw that the whole rose was made up of many different parts: the roots that anchor the flower and collect the nutrients, the stems that support the heads, the flowers that attract the bees, the leaves that absorb the sunlight, and also the thorns that protect the whole plant. Each of these physical aspects also has a function. I then started to think about the human body, and I started to get overwhelmed. All the different parts of the body that exist, and all the functions that need to happen for the body to live; it seems like it is impossible to grasp."

Grandmother Terra understood Sun's feeling of being overwhelmed by the complexity of the human body. She had had the same feeling when she started her studies and saw a bit of herself in her grandchild. "Yes, Sun. The human body is vast in its functions and forms. Yet there is a logic that can help us understand it. Just like to understand nature we use the five elements to help make sense of the totality of our environment, we do the same for the body. We use the internal organs to classify the functions and how they interact with each other."

Sun understood. "OK. There are so many organs, though; how can we understand all of them?"

Grandfather Terra chuckled. "Indeed, Sun. There are many physical organs in the body. However, in Chinese medicine we simplify it a bit. We take a total of ten physical organs and two non-physical organs and assign all the functions of the body to these 12 organs. It is a kind of classification system, like the five elements.

"The internal organs are divided into two separate groups, a Yin group and a Yang group. The Yang group are mainly related to the ingestion, digestion, and elimination of liquids and solids. The Yin group is more about how the Qi that is extracted from the solids and liquids are used in the body. The Yin group also deals with the gases that enter the body, such as air.

"Let's start by thinking of the Yang organs and the way we digest food according to Chinese medicine. The food and liquid enter the body through the mouth and descend to the Stomach. So the Stomach is the first Yang organ. The Stomach ripens and breaks down the food. It starts the process of extracting the nutrients from the food and transforming them into Qi. The Stomach uses the bile in the Gall Bladder to help break down the fats. So the Gall Bladder is the second Yang organ. The ripened food and liquid then continue to the Small Intestine. Here the Small Intestine starts separating the pure Qi that is still in the solids from the unrefined Qi that the body does not need. The Small Intestine is the third Yang organ.

"Once all the Qi that can be extracted from the food and drink is extracted, it sends the solids to the Large Intestine and the liquid to the Bladder. The Large Intestine takes the solids and starts to move them toward the exterior of the body. Before it finally pushes the unwanted solids from the body it takes out the last of the liquid and sends it to the Bladder. The Large Intestine is the fourth Yang channel. And finally, the Bladder takes the unwanted liquid from the Small Intestine and the Large Intestine and pushes it out of the body. The Bladder is the fifth Yang organ. So, the Yang organs are the Stomach, Gall Bladder, Small Intestine, Large Intestine, and Bladder. Here I have only talked about their main functions. They have many more functions, but for understanding the big picture that is enough for now."

Sun responded, "OK. So there are five Yang organs, and they're all involved in taking in or getting rid of food and drink. They all take in and can get full, and then can be empty again waiting for the next batch of food and drink. They process the Qi from the food and drink. Where does this Qi go?"

"Good summary and question," responded Grandmother Terra. "The Qi goes to the Yin organs for them to refine and use in the body. There are five Yin organs, and their flow is not as linear as that of the Yang organs. They have many more interactions and joint processes than the Yang organs. The Yin organs are the Heart, Lung, Spleen, Liver, and Kidneys. The main function of the Lung is taking in the air and extracting what the body needs from the air, which we call oxygen. The Spleen, which also includes the idea of the pancreas, takes the transformed Qi from the Yang organs and refines it for the rest of the body to use. The Heart is mainly responsible for sending the Qi-rich blood around the body. It is also important in the spiritual and emotional functions of the body. The Liver's main function is to ensure the smooth flow of Qi throughout the body. Finally, there are the Kidneys. They are the most internal organ and stock the refined substances that the body needs. They are also related to reproduction and other long cycles. This is just a very brief summary. The study of internal organs is vast, and we do not have time for that here."

"OK," replied Sun. "There are five Yang and five Yin organs. The Yang organs are more exterior, and the Yin organs are more internal. This means the Yin organs deal with more refined and treated Qi. As the Qi is refined and the body can use it, they can stock the Qi, and as the Qi is refined, they cannot be full. Is that the idea?"

"Woohoo," Grandfather Terra tooted unexpectedly. "You got it kid, those are the important points about the Yin and Yang organs. More tea, Sun?" Grandfather Terra was already filling up Sun's cup.

Laughing, Sun thanked their grandfather for the tea. "I've realized that there is always a structure and logic to Chinese medicine. I find it interesting that there are five Yin organs, five Yang organs, and five elements. If I am not mistaken, each Yin organ can be associated with a Yang organ and an element. So, each element would have a Yin and Yang organ. I know that these associations are mentioned in the classics, but I just don't see the logic of the associations. Could you explain this to me?"

Grandmother Terra smiled. "Of course we can explain it. We are teachers, after all. To understand the associations, we need to look at the physical organs and Yin and Yang. First, let's start by looking at the Yin organs, because the Yin organs are the key points that all the associations revolve around. There are five Yin organs: the Heart, the Lungs, the Spleen, the Liver, and the Kidneys. If we look at where these organs are in the body, we will find that they are all between the collarbone and the umbilicus line (where your belly button is). Now, if we take the mid-distance between these two limits, the collarbone and the umbilicus line, we have the diaphragm. Above the diaphragm there is the Heart and the Lungs, and below the diaphragm there is the Spleen, Liver, and Kidneys. Using the Yin Yang approach, we could say that the Heart and Lungs are more Yang as they are above the diaphragm and closer to the sun, and the Spleen, Liver, and Kidneys are more Yin as they are below the diaphragm. So, within the group of Yin organs we have two that are more Yang and three that are more Yin. The two organs that are more Yang we will associate with elements that are more Yang, and the three that are more Yin we will associate with the elements that are more Yin.

"So, let's look at the elements again.

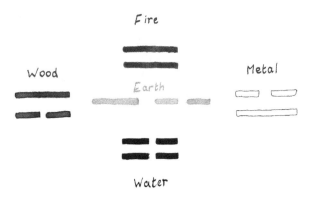

"The elements where the bottom line is solid are more Yang elements, and where the bottom line is broken are more Yin elements. The earth element, which has both a solid and a broken line, is considered more Yin because it is called earth, and that is the opposite of heaven, which makes it more Yin.

"We have two Yang elements, fire and metal, and three Yin elements, earth, wood, and water. Now let's associate the Yin organs that are above the diaphragm with the elements that are more Yang. We can use many associations of the elements to decide how we categorize the organs. For fire and metal, let's look at colors. Fire is red and metal is white. If we look at the organs, the Heart is red, and the Lungs are white. We will associate the Heart with fire and the Lungs with metal.

"Now for the Yin organs below the diaphragm and the elements that are more Yin. Earth is the center, and is the element that has the most transformation associated with it. It is the transitionary interseason. Of the three lower Yin organs, this is like the Spleen, with its function of transforming the Qi from food into useful Qi for the body. The Spleen is associated with earth.

"Wood is like a tree. It has its roots deep below the earth, so it is rooted in Yin and grows tall above the earth, so it manifests itself as Yang. A tree grows upward and outward. This is like the Liver's function of sending Qi all around the body. So for this reason, the Liver is associated with wood.

"Water is the most Yin of the elements. As the element suggests, it is associated with the organ that has the most to do with internal liquids, like urine for example. It is obvious that this is the Kidneys as they filter the urine. So, the Kidneys are associated with water."

Sun wanted to make sure they got it all so far. "OK. Each of the five elements will have a Yin and Yang organ. The Yin organs are the key to the associations, and this is somewhat based on where they are in the body in relation to the other Yin organs. If the Yin organ is above the diaphragm, it is associated with an element that is more rooted in Yang, and if it is below the diaphragm it is associated with an element that is more rooted in Yin. We can use the functions of the organ or the color of the organ to find the associated element.

"Just an idea—could we also use the placement of the organs to associate with the elements? We could put the elements in a line from most Yin to most Yang. Moving up from the bottom of the torso, we first find Kidney, which is the most Yin and so water, then there is the Liver and wood, next is the Spleen and earth, then the Lungs and metal, and the final organ of the Heart with fire."

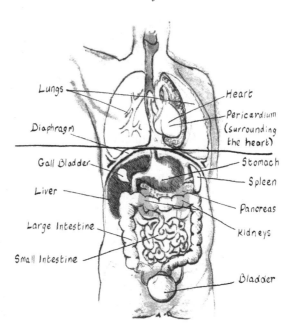

"Very good, Sun," replied Grandfather Terra. "That is also a way to understand the associations. And then we must add the Yang organs to the associations. We will use their physical placements in the body to do this. Let's start by looking at the Yin element/organ pairs.

"The three Yin elements and the associated organs that are below the diaphragm all have a physical connection to the Yang organ they are associated with. The Liver is connected to the Gall Bladder, the Kidneys are connected to the Bladder, and the Pancreas (which is part of the Spleen in Chinese medicine) is connected to the Stomach. So, the Yin elements with their associated organs are:

Wood—Liver—Gall Bladder

Water—Kidneys—Bladder

Earth—Spleen—Stomach.

"For the Yin organs above the diaphragm, Heart and Lungs, they do not physically connect to their Yang organs. However, there is a different type of connection. They are images of each other."

Sun wasn't sure what that meant. "What do you mean by images of each other?"

"What I mean is that there is a physical similarity in their positioning and form that allows them to be associated. First, look at where they are situated in the body. The Lungs and the Heart are both above the diaphragm, and the Small Intestine and the Large Intestine are both situated below the umbilicus. The Yin organs are in the most upper part of the torso, and the Yang organs are in the lower part of the torso, with neither in the middle part of the torso. And now look at their position relative to the other organs around them. The Heart is in the middle of the chest and is surrounded by the Lungs, and the Small Intestine is in the middle of the lower abdomen and is surrounded by the Large Intestine. Look at the following picture."

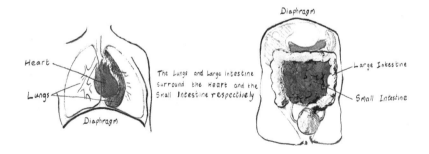

The Lungs and Large Intestine surround the Heart and the Small Intestine respectively

Sun got what his grandfather was saying. When put in relation to the other organ, they are images of each other.

Grandmother Terra added, "Also, if you look at how the organs move, they are similar. The Heart makes strong and powerful contractions to pump the blood all over the body, and the Small Intestine makes strong, tight contractions to move the food along, whereas the Lungs expand and contract much more slowly but have more change from when they are full to when they are empty; the Large Intestine has similar movements to help move the stool out of the body. Therefore, we say the following:

Fire—Heart—Small Intestine

Metal—Lungs—Large Intestine.

Sun thought he got it all. "OK. There are five elements, five Yin organs, and five Yang organs. *Organ* refers to the physical tissue that is in the body and all the functions that are assigned to it. The Yang organs' functions are more related to the ingestion, digestion, and elimination of food and liquids, and the Yin organs are more related to taking the Qi that the Yang organs extract from the food and drink and using it to nourish and make the rest of the body function.

"To associate the organs with the elements we use the position of the Yin organs as our guide. We take the elements and classify them from the most Yang to the most Yin:

Fire—Metal—Earth—Wood—Water.

"We then take the Yin organs and look at their position in the body, going from the thorax down to the umbilicus. We take the lowest point of each organ and put them in the same order as the elements:

Heart—Lungs—Spleen—Liver—Kidneys.

"Finally, for the Yang organs there are two different reasons for associating them with a Yin organ. For the Yin organs that are below the diaphragm there is a physical connection between the Yin and Yang organs. For the Yin organs above the diaphragm and the Yang organs below the umbilicus, we use the relationship of the Heart to the Lungs and the Small Intestine to the Large Intestine, the similarities they share in placement, and the way they expand and contract.

"This gives a final association grouping of:

Fire—Heart—Small Intestine

Metal—Lungs—Large Intestine

Earth—Spleen—Stomach

Wood—Liver—Gall Bladder

Water—Kidneys—Bladder."

All three looked at each other smiling, knowing that Sun got it. And knowing that it was enough for today.

13

THE THREE DIVISIONS OF THE HUMAN BODY

Sun spent the next day mulling over all they had learned so far. They thought about Yin and Yang, the five elements, and Qi. It all seemed magical and logical at the same time. They had already been with their grandparents a while, and they still hadn't really talked about what Sun was most interested in.

Sun waited until they were sitting on the porch drinking the tea Grandmother Terra had made, and then they dove right in. "I have really enjoyed our talks and lessons these last few weeks. Yet I'm starting to notice some anxiety in myself that we have not really talked about what I thought we were going to study this summer. I was expecting to study the channels of the body."

Sipping her tea and looking at Sun, Grandmother Terra smiled. "Sun, we have been discussing the channels from the beginning. Traditionally the channels were taught by memorizing them, with no explanation as to why they are where they are. Your grandfather and I realized long ago that this was not the best way to understand and learn about the channels. Everything we've been talking about is going to help us to understand the channels without memorizing them. We've been giving you the foundations upon which channels are built. With that said, we are now ready to start exploring the channels in more detail.

"First, do you remember what we said a channel is?"

"A channel has two meanings. The first is a vertical segment of the body that helps us understand where we are on the body. The second is that the vertical segment is filled with Qi, and that it flows within the segment," Sun said proudly.

Grandmother Terra laughed. "Very good, teacher's pet. We will concentrate on the vertical segments for the moment. You can think of the body as eight cylinders over four parts of the body. The body is first divided into two separate parts, the left side and the right side. The left side has one cylinder for the head, one for the body, one for the arm, and one for the leg.

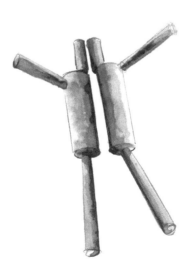

"If we see the totality like this, we have two main aspects, the limbs and the body. The limbs are made up of the arms and the legs, and the body is made up of the torso and the head. We also have a left side and a right side. The right and left sides are completely symmetric. This means that when we study the channels, whatever we say about the right side of the body we say also about the left side. So, when we talk about a channel, it will be present on the right side as well as the left side and occupy the same space."

Sun responded, "So it is like the muscles and bones. What is on the left side is also on the right side. All the bones and muscles are the same on the right side of the body and the left side. The channels are the same."

"Exactly," chimed in Grandfather Terra. "When we talk about a channel, it will exist on both sides of the body. Now, the next point to understand is that the limbs, arms and legs, are divided slightly differently than the body. The limbs are first divided into Yin and Yang. As we said before, the part that gets the most amount of sun is the Yang side, and the part that gets the least amount of sun is the Yin side. The torso and the head are not separated in the same way.

"So far, we have four cylinders on the right side and four on the left. If we just look at the right side for now, two are the limbs and two are the body. The limbs are first divided into Yin and Yang. We are then going to divide each cylinder into three segments, front, middle, and back.

"Here is a cross section of an arm where the thumb is pointing up. The top of the arm is the front section, and has a Yang part and a Yin part which are next to each other. The middle has a Yang part and Yin part that are opposite each other. On your forearm this will be between the two bones, the radius and the ulna bones. The back part is like the front part, as the Yin and Yang side are touching.

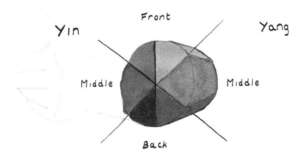

"On the arm there are three areas that are Yin and three areas that are Yang. The side of the arm in line with the palm is the Yin side, and it is divided into front, middle, and back. The opposite side of the arm, in line with the back of the hand, is Yang and is divided into front, middle, and back.

"The arm has six sections. Each section has two components: Yin/Yang and front, middle, or back.

"If we say front Yin on the hand, that is the fleshy muscle on the palm of the hand near the thumb. And if we say front Yang on the hand, that is the back of the hand between the thumb and the index finger.

"The middle Yin of the forearm is on the palm side of the arm and between the two tendons. The Yang middle is on the back of the forearm between the two bones.

"Finally, the back Yin at the wrist is on the palm side where the little finger line meets the wrist. The back Yang is also where the little finger line meets the wrist, but on the back of the hand."

Sun observed, "When you say front, middle, and back it is making reference to swinging my arms next to my body when I walk. The front is the part that is closest to the sun when I swing the arm forward. The back is the side closest to the sun when I swing my arm back. And the middle is between the two."

"Exactly," confirmed Grandmother Terra. "Those are the

three divisions of the arm, and each division has a Yang side and a Yin side.

"The leg follows the same logic. There is a Yang side and a Yin side, and a front, middle, and back division. We separate the Yin and Yang on the leg by going down from the hip, over the kneecap, and over the front of the foot.

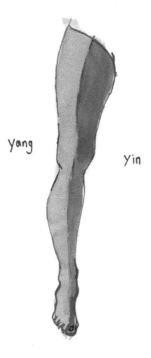

yang

yin

"If we use the knee to define the divisions, the kneecap is the front, the sides of the knee between the bone and the tendons are the middle, and the crease in the back is the back.

"So just like the arm and the leg, we have a Yin side and a Yang side. And we have three divisions, front, middle, and back. There is a front Yin and a front Yang which are next to each other. They cover the front of the thigh. There is the middle Yin, which is on the interior of the leg, and a middle Yang, which is on the exterior of the leg. When you are wearing jeans, the seam of the jeans leg is the middle Yin and Yang. Finally, there is the back Yin and back Yang. This is where the hamstrings are, on the thigh."

Sun got it. "The arms and the legs both have a Yin side and a Yang side. When walking normally with the arms hanging by the body and the palm almost touching the leg, the front division is the part that when moving forward actually moves forward. The back division is the part of the arm exposed to the sun when the arm swings back, and the part exposed to the sun on the leg that is moving back relative to the body. The middle is the part that is in the middle."

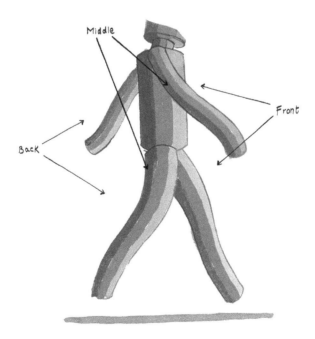

Grandfather Terra nodded approvingly. "Very good, Sun, that's it. Now, when it comes to the body and the head, we do not first separate the cylinder into Yin and Yang. We have a front division, middle division, and back division, and then in the front section we have a Yin segment and a Yang segment. We won't describe this yet though. It will make more sense when we talk about each different cylinder individually.

"So, what we have is that there are Yin segments and Yang segments. There are front, middle, and back segments. With these two pieces of information, we have six segments for each cylinder. Every cylinder has the same number of Yin segments and the same number of Yang segments. Every cylinder also has the same number of front, middle, and back segments. Now, instead of using the word *segment*, we will use the word *channel*. So, the foot has six channels, three Yin and three Yang, two in the front, two in the middle, and two in the back. The arm also has six channels, three that are Yin and three that are Yang, two in the front, two in the middle, and two in the back.

"There are six channels in the foot and six in the arm. How many channels are there on one side of the body?"

Sun replied excitedly, "Twelve channels, six in the arm and six in the foot. In the arm there are three Yin channels and three Yang. The three Yin channels are front, middle, and back, and the three Yang channels are also front, middle, and back. The same is true for the foot. So the names of the 12 channels could be:

Arm front Yin

Arm middle Yin

Arm back Yin

Arm front Yang

Arm middle Yang

Arm back Yang

Foot front Yin

Foot middle Yin

Foot back Yin

Foot front Yang

Foot middle Yang

Foot back Yang.

"But what about the body and the head? Don't they also have channels?"

"The channels in the body and the head use the channels of the hands and feet. So there are 12 channels, just like you said. And we could use the positions for the names, but each channel has a different name. That is what we will talk about tomorrow."

Sun knew teatime had finished for that day.

PART IV

UNDERSTANDING OF THE CHANNELS

14

THE GENERAL FLOW
OF CHANNELS

The next day, teatime could not come soon enough, but it eventually came. To make it come quicker, Sun offered to help make the tea. Grandfather Terra was delighted and showed Sun the intricate and complex way he made it, following the traditional way of making tea for a tea ceremony. When Sun asked if all the preparation and multiple steps made a difference to the flavor he just laughed, and started pouring the tea without answering. Sun understood that it didn't matter if the tea tasted better, it was the ritual that he enjoyed, like Sun learning about Chinese medicine and the channels. Regardless of whether they would use them, the effort of learning was a reward in itself.

All three gathered on the porch and sipped the tea, which tasted the same as if it had been made differently, and yet enjoying it more because it was made with intention. After a few sips, Sun started with a new question. "Yesterday we finally started to see the channels in a way that covers the whole body. They are starting to come to life for me. We said that a channel has two meanings: a geographical vertical segment of the body, which is what we saw yesterday, and also a channel or conduit in which the Qi flows. Can you help me understand better how the Qi flows?"

Grandfather Terra responded, "Yes, that is the second function of the channel—to be a place where Qi moves. The movement of Qi, like everything else, is based on Yin and Yang. As we have said many times, Yang is the sun and the heavens in relation to Yin, which is the earth. The human body is between heaven and earth.

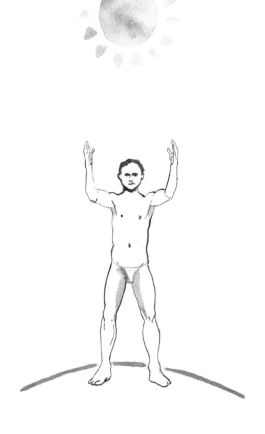

"The sun, which is above and is Yang, comes down toward the earth. So, Yang will have a downward movement. The earth, which is below and is Yin, moves up toward the sun. So, Yin will have an upward movement.

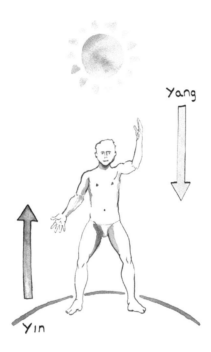

"When we think about how the channels flow, it is good to picture a person with their hands above their heads. Their hands are the closest to the sun, so the Yang Qi will first arrive there and then make its way down to the head and from the head down to the feet.

"The feet are the closest to the earth, so the Yin Qi will start in the feet and move up to the chest, and then from the chest out to the hands."

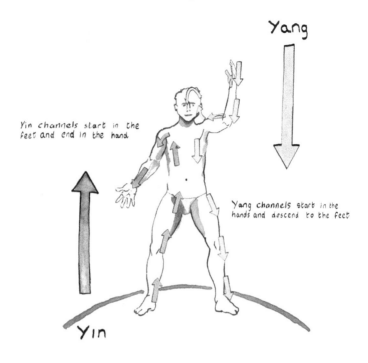

Yang

Yin channels start in the feet and end in the hand

Yang channels start in the hands and descend to the feet

Yin

Sun wanted to make sure they understood. "So, as the sun is more Yang in relation to the earth, which is more Yin, the Qi that comes down from above is more Yang. And as the earth is more Yin in relation to the sun, which is more Yang, the Qi that comes up from the earth is more Yin. In other words, Yin Qi starts in the feet and moves upward, and the Yang Qi starts in the hands and moves downward. What happens when the Yang Qi gets all the way to the feet? Does it just stop?"

Grandmother Terra was happy to respond. "At the feet, a Yang channel will move its Qi to a Yin channel and the Qi will flow upward. And at the hands, where the Yin Qi has moved all the way up through the body, the Yin Qi will change polarity and move to a Yang channel. The word *polarity* here means either Yin or Yang.

"So at the extremities, the Qi changes polarity. In the feet, it changes from Yang to Yin, and in the hands, it changes from Yin to Yang."

Sun was excited. "So there is a constant flow in the channels. The Yin Qi flows down from the hands to the feet and changes polarity to Yin channels, and then flows back up to the hands where it changes again. It's like a circle that never stops."

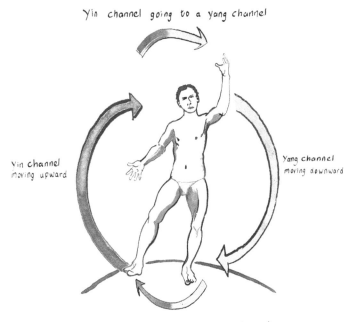

Yin channel going to a yang channel

Yin channel moving upward

Yang channel moving downward

Yang channel going to a yin channel

"Very good," replied Grandfather Terra. "So, there is a constant cycle of Qi running through the body and alternating from Yin to Yang channels. To really understand the flow, we need to add one more piece of information. The Yang Qi moves from the hand down to the head and further down to the foot. The Yin Qi moves from the foot up to the thorax, and then out to the hand. One full movement from either the hand to the foot or the foot to the hand follows the same division that we already talked about. You remember front, middle, and back?"

"Of course I do," said Sun. "And I also remember you saying that each division was separated into two different parts, the arm and the foot. How does that come into this whole picture?"

Grandmother Terra was happy with the question. "That is what helps us complete and create the cycle. Each division is separated into two parts, a foot and a hand part. And how we define the foot and hand part depends on the polarity—if the channel is Yin or Yang.

"For the Yang segment, the part of the channel that goes from the hand to the head is called the hand channel, and the segment that goes from the head to the foot is called the foot channel. For the Yin segments, the part that goes from the foot to the thorax or upper body is the foot segment, and the part that goes from the upper body to the hand is the hand segment.

"We could say that the Yang channels meet in the head and the Yin channels meet in the upper body. In a picture it would look like this."

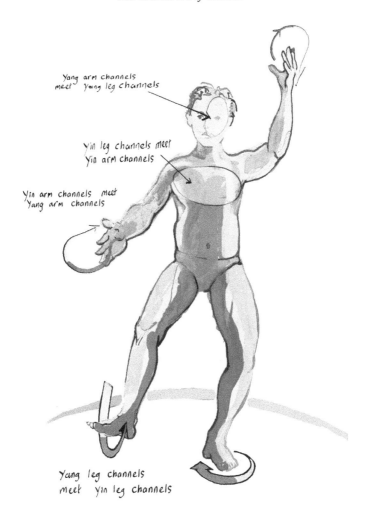

Yang arm channels
meet Yang leg channels

Yin leg channels meet
Yin arm channels

Yin arm channels meet
Yang arm channels

Yang leg channels
meet yin leg channels

Sun saw it now. "So, it is a constant cycle of four different parts. We have Yin and Yang and arm and foot. And they are constantly interacting and changing with each other. Each transition will either be a transition between a foot and hand channel or a Yin and Yang channel. The transition from Yin to Yang happens in the hand, and the transition from Yang to Yin happens in the foot. The Yin channels transition from foot to hand in the upper body and the Yang channels transition from hand to foot in the head.

"We could start the cycle anywhere and it will always bring us back to the same place. For example, let's start in the upper body. The channel that starts in the upper body is a Yin arm channel. The Qi will flow from the upper body out to the hand. Here it will change its polarity and follow the Yang channel. The Qi will flow up the hand to the head, and in the head it will transfer from the hand Yang channel to the foot Yang channel. The foot Yang channel will flow down the body toward the foot, and in the foot the Qi will change polarity and move to a Yin channel. The Yin foot channel will flow back up all the way to the upper body, finishing where we started in the upper body. And from there again it will go to a hand Yin channel and flow out to the hand."

"That is exactly it," Grandmother Terra said with some pride in her voice. "And by chance you chose the best example by starting in the upper body, the reason being that each segment, front, middle, or back, starts in the upper body. The Qi will go through the cycle of hand Yin to hand Yang to foot Yang to foot Yin all in one continuous flow. When it gets back to the upper body it will then change its position and do the cycle again. The order it does this in is the front segments, then the back segments, then the middle segments, and then back to the front segments."

"OK, I see this flow now. Each channel has a polarity (Yin or Yang), a limb (hand or foot), and a position (front, middle, or back). The polarity determines the direction the Qi flows in, the limb defines which part of the channel we are talking about, and the position gives the order to the flow."

"Great," said Grandfather Terra. "Now let's enjoy the rest of the tea."

It had been a good day.

15

THE MEANING BEHIND THE CHINESE NAMES OF THE CHANNELS

Another peaceful and active day passed, working in the garden and going for a pleasant walk. The routine was pleasant, and Sun now understood why their grandparents were taking time to explain things to them. By learning in chunks, Sun was able to understand what they were learning. They were enthralled with the channels and wanted to go further.

Once the tea was served, Sun started once again. "In the classics and the other books I have read, the channels have long names. They're not called by their position but have Chinese words and organs in their names. Can you please explain this to me?"

Grandmother Terra smiled. "Of course we can. Like all things in Chinese medicine, there is a logic and meaning, and channel names are no different. The answer is that the Chinese names describe the amount of sun each vertical segment gets and which parts of the body it refers to. Each name has four components:

The first component is whether it is situated in the hand or foot.

The second component is how much sun it gets.

The third component is whether it is on the Yin or Yang side of the body.

The final component is the organ that is associated with it.

"Let's start by looking at the first three components, and leave the organ associations to another time. We saw that each cylinder is divided into three divisions: front, middle, and back. The legs and the arms are also divided into Yin and Yang. The torso also has Yin and Yang, but the three divisions of front, middle, and back come first. We can also add that the head only has Yang channels, as it is the most Yang part of the body."

Sun jumped in. "I was wondering about that. We didn't really talk about the torso and the head yesterday. Why did we jump over it?"

Grandfather Terra responded, "The arms and legs are easier to understand, and they help us get the general logic. The torso has a slightly different logic, and so does the head. So we start by understanding the easier logic first and then build up to the more complex."

"OK. That makes sense. Sorry, please continue Grandmother," responded Sun.

"As I was saying," continued Grandmother Terra. "We have three components that we will look at for the moment. The first component is the arm or the leg. This is telling us where the channel starts or finishes. As we saw yesterday, the arm Yin channels start in the torso and finish in the hand, the arm Yang channels start in the hand and finish in the head, the foot Yang channels start in the head and finish in the foot, and finally the foot Yin channels start in the foot and finish in the torso.

"The next aspect is the Chinese name that is associated with the channel. There are four different Chinese words that can be associated with a channel. These words are:

Tai

Shao

Ming

Jue.

"And these names refer to the amount of sun the position of the channel gets in relation to the other channels. I know that sounds confusing, but let us break it down and it will become clearer. Remember that Chinese words can have many different meanings depending on how they are used. In relation to the channels, each word is referring to the quantity of the sunlight.

"There are three positions on the Yang side of the body (front, middle, and back) and three positions on the Yin side of the body (front, middle, and back). Each position on the Yang part of the body is exposed to a different amount of sunlight. One will get the most amount of sunlight, one will get a medium amount of sunlight, and one will get the least amount of sunlight. The same is true on the Yin side.

"We use *Tai*, which means greater, to describe the segment that gets the most amount of sunlight. For example, on the Yang aspect of the body, the segment that gets the most amount of sunlight is the back. The back of the torso and the back of the arms receive the most sunlight on the body. So the back-Yang position is called Tai Yang."

Sun interrupted. "Hold on. Why does the back get the most sun? If I'm standing straight wouldn't the sun touch all places equally?"

Grandfather Terra smiled. "Well, not exactly. And also,

we rarely stand directly upright. In fact, whenever we walk or do any activity we are always slightly bent forward. This is especially true when we are gardening, farming, or doing any activity. When humans are outside, we are usually slightly bent forward. The best position to imagine when understanding how much sunlight a part of the body gets is the position of working in a field—either bending over to dig, or crouching and slightly bent over to pick something up.

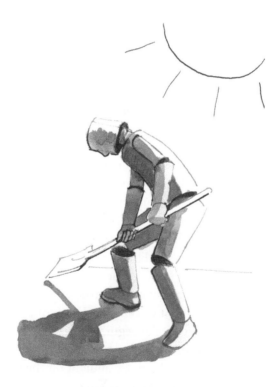

"Here you can see that when we are in this position, most of the sunlight is on the back, and the back of the arms and the legs get more sun than the front of the arms and legs.

"The next position on the Yang side to get the second-most amount of sunlight is the front position.

"*Ming* means bright in Chinese, and as this gets the second-most amount of sunlight, we call this the Yang Ming—the reason this word is used comes from the Chinese clock, which we will explain later. The reason we put Yang in front of the word Ming is because of Chinese grammar; in all the other cases we put the Chinese word in front of the Yin or Yang. When we are talking about channels, Ming represents the medium amount of sunlight on the Yang side.

"That leaves the middle segment on the Yang side. This segment gets the least amount of sunlight. On the torso it is covered by the arms, and on the limbs, it has the most shadows as it is protected from the sun. For the least amount of sunlight, we call it *Shao*. Shao means lesser. So, we say Shao Yang gets the least amount of sunlight on the Yang side of the body.

"For the Yang segments we have:

Back—most sunlight—Tai Yang

Front—medium sunlight—Yang Ming

Middle—least sunlight—Shao Yang.

"The Yin side has a different order. The area on the Yin side that gets the most amount of sunlight is the front, so the front segment is called Tai Yin. *Tai* means most sunlight, and *Yin* means on the Yin side.

"The segment that gets the medium amount of sunlight is the middle Yin segment. This is called Jue Yin. *Jue* means terminal, and like *Ming*, the name comes from the Chinese clock.

"The back segment of the Yin side gets the least amount of sunlight and is called Shao Yin. *Shao* here means the least amount of sunlight on the Yin side.

"If we put it all together it would look like this:

Amount of Sunlight	Chinese Name	Position on Limb
Most on Yin channel	Tai Yin	Front
Medium on Yin channel	Jue Yin	Middle
Least on Yin channel	Shao Yin	Back
Most on Yang channel	Tai Yang	Back
Medium on Yang channel	Yang Ming	Front
Least on Yang channel	Shao Yang	Middle

"And if we drew it on the arm it would look like this."

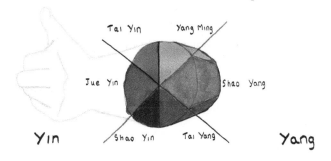

Sun responded, "Let me see if I have got this straight. The Chinese names tell us four pieces of information: the part of the body the channel either starts or finishes in (foot or hand); whether the segment is on the Yin or Yang side of the body; the amount of sunlight that segment gets in relation to the other segments of the same Yin or Yang side; and finally the organ that is associated with it—which we will see later.

"The Chinese word *Tai* means most amount of sunlight, *Shao* means the least amount of sunlight, and the words *Jue* and *Ming* mean a medium amount of sunlight. The names *Jue* and *Ming* you will explain later when we see the Chinese clock.

"The Yin side of the body and the Yang side of the body have different orders in the amount of sun they get.

"On the Yang side:

Most amount of sunlight—back

Medium amount of sunlight—front

Least amount of sunlight—middle.

"So, the back Yang channel is called Tai Yang, the front Yang channel is called Yang Ming, and the middle Yang channel is called Shao Yang.

"The order of the Yin channels in relation to the sunlight is different:

Most amount of sunlight—front

Medium amount of sunlight—middle

Least amount of sunlight—back.

"So the front Yin channel is called Tai Yin, the middle Yin channel is called Jue Yin, and the back Yin channel is called Shao Yin."

Grandmother Terra smiled. "You got it. And it is important to understand the last bit of the channel names, which is the organ associated with the channel. We will see that tomorrow as I am hungry, and your grandfather has promised us a nice meal this evening."

All their stomachs were telling them they were hungry, and it was dinnertime. The organs would wait until tomorrow.

16

ASSOCIATING THE
ORGANS AND BOWELS
WITH THE CHANNELS

Another pleasant day passed. Sun had learned to enjoy the part of the day when they were not learning. Taking the time to integrate what they had learned the day before and putting it into context was deepening their understanding of their knowledge. Sun was still excited for that day's lesson, but with less impatience. They had accepted that there is a time for acquiring information and a time for quiet, and the time for quiet was just as important. Sun laughed to themselves, thinking, "I have also learned the meaning of patience."

It was teatime for the trio. Sun asked if they could serve the tea today, and the grandparents accepted Sun's offer with smiles on their faces. They were so pleased at seeing their grandchild blossoming. After the tea was served Sun sat down, took a sip, and looked at their grandparents. They were ready for today's talk.

Sun started, "We talked about how the names of the channels have many components: the placement of the channel (foot or hand), the polarity of the channel (Yin or Yang), and the Chinese name for the amount of sunlight it receives. From reading the classics, I think there is still one aspect that we have not discussed yet. Each channel also has an organ in its name. We talked about the five Yin organs and the five Yang organs, yet there are six Yin channels and six Yang channels. I feel like we are missing some information. Can you please talk to me about how the organs are associated with the channels, and what the two extra organs are that we have not talked about yet?"

Grandmother Terra nodded. "Indeed, you have made a good observation, Sun. This is one of the sticking points in Chinese medicine, and perhaps to understand it we need to add a bit of context. Chinese medicine and philosophy were not developed in a continuous timeline where each development was based on the previous. The five-element school of thought was connected to the channel system after it had been developed. That meant that the use of five elements to explain the environment was independent of Chinese medicine during its development, and was incorporated at a later point. And this separate development led to one major problem when using the 12 channels: How to put the five elements with their associated organs with the channels. We will attempt to explain how this is done in as simple a way as possible.

"First, we will use the five Yin and five Yang organs that we have already talked about, and then we will introduce the new organs and talk about how they can be included in the five element system.

"When we talk about associating organs with channels, we will use the Yin organs as our guide, and the Yang organs will follow. Let's start with the five Yin organs: the Kidneys, Liver, Spleen, Lungs, and Heart. We had associated them with the elements by looking at their physical placement in the body and connecting that placement to the Yin/Yang dynamic of each element. The most Yin element (water) is associated with the lowest Yin organ (Kidneys), and the most Yang element (fire) is associated with the organ that is highest in the body (Heart). Then we associated the Lungs with metal, the Liver with wood, and the Spleen with earth. So, let us look at these five Yin organs and how we place them on the channels.

"All the Yin organs are situated between the collarbone and the belly button. Halfway between these two points is the diaphragm. Any organ that is above the diaphragm is more Yang in relation to the organs below the diaphragm. Therefore, the organs above the diaphragm are associated with channels in the arms, and the organs below the diaphragm are associated with channels in the legs."

Sun thought he got it. "That would mean that the Heart and Lungs are associated with arm channels as they are above the diaphragm, and the Kidneys, Liver, and Spleen are in the legs as they are below the diaphragm."

"Exactly," chimed in Grandfather Terra. "So far we have two organs that are associated with the arm channels and three organs associated with the leg channels. Let's look at the leg channels now. We have the Kidneys, Liver, and Spleen. We have Tai, Jue, and Shao Yin, or most amount of sunlight, medium amount of sunlight, and least amount of sunlight, or front position, middle position, and back position. The way we now associate the organs with the channels is by looking at the organ function and how much it interacts with the external world. The organ that has the most interaction with the external world and the most sunlight will be in the front, Tai Yin. The organ that has the medium amount of interaction with the exterior world and medium sunlight will be in the middle, Jue Yin. And finally, the organ that interacts the least with the external world and has the least sunlight will be associated with the back, Shao Yin."

Sun was nodding and seeing the logic. "We didn't talk a lot about the organs' functions in Chinese medicine. Yet what I think I understood is that of the three organs that are below the diaphragm, the Spleen would have the most interaction with the external world as it takes the Qi from the Stomach and transforms it into Qi for the rest of the body to use. So I guess that would mean that the Front Foot Tai Yin channel is the Spleen."

"Perfect, Sun. You got it," Grandmother Terra beamed. "Now, between the Liver and the Kidney, which one has less contact with the external world?"

Sun thought for a moment. "I think it is the Kidney. I remember the Kidneys are the deepest of the Yin organs and also the lowest in the body. I think the Kidneys are associated with the Back Foot Shao Yin channel. And that would leave the Middle Foot Jue Yin channel to the Liver. Is that correct?"

"That is correct," responded Grandfather Terra. "Now let's couple them with their associated Yang organs. The Yin organ that is associated with a position on the leg will have the Yang organ that it shares the element with in the same position, but on the Yang side. So, we have Kidney in the back on the Shao Yin channel of the foot. The Kidney is associated with water, and the Yang organ associated with water is the Bladder. Therefore, the Bladder will be on the back Tai Yang foot position."

"OK," said Sun. "I think I get it. Let me try to apply the same logic to the other Yin leg channels. We put the Liver on the middle position of the Yin side of the leg. We called this position Jue Yin. The Liver is associated with the element of wood. The Yang organ in the wood element is the Gall Bladder. So, the middle position on the Yang side of the leg that is called Foot Shao Yang will also have the Gall Bladder associated with it. Is that correct?"

"That is perfect," smiled Grandfather Terra.

Sun continued, "The last leg channel is the front position. We put the Spleen on the Yin side on the Foot Tai Yin channel. The Spleen is associated with the earth element. The Yang organ also associated with earth is the Stomach. So, the front Yang Ming channel is associated with the Stomach.

"So, the names of the channels of the leg and their positions are:

Front position: Foot Tai Yin Spleen on the Yin side and Foot Yang Ming Stomach on the Yang side.

Middle position: Foot Jue Yin Liver on the Yin side and Foot Shao Yang Gall Bladder on the Yang side.

Back position: Foot Shao Yin Kidney on the Yin side and Foot Tai Yang Bladder on the Yang side."

"That is exactly it," replied Grandmother Terra. "Now, when we look at the channels themselves, we will see that there are some particular features of the leg as to the positions, but you nailed it.

"Now the arm channels are slightly more complicated, because we only have two Yin organs that have yet to be associated and three Yin channels on the arm. And the same is true for the Yang channels.

"The last two elements that we have not used are the two Yang-based elements, metal and fire, and their associated Yin organs are the Lungs and the Heart. We said that the Yin organs above the diaphragm are the Yin organs associated with the arm Yin channels. If we look at the human body, there are no other major organs that are between the collarbone and the diaphragm. However, there is an important membrane that goes all around the Heart, which is called the Pericardium. The Pericardium protects the Heart. This is the last Yin organ that we use to complete the Yin organs.

"We now have three Yin organs above the diaphragm—

the Lungs, Heart, and Pericardium—and three Yin channels on the arm—Front Tai Yin, Middle Jue Yin, and Back Shao Yin. To associate the organs with the channels we will apply the same logic as we did with the foot channels and Yin organs."

Sun replied, "I get it. We look at which organ has the most interaction with the exterior and match that organ to the channel that gets the most amount of sunlight. We then do the same for the middle organ and the middle amount of sunlight, and again for the least amount of sunlight and the organ with the least amount of contact with the exterior.

"I think the organ that is in contact with the exterior the most out of the three Yin organs above the diaphragm is the Lungs. They take in the air and the air comes from the exterior. I would say that the Lungs go with the front arm channel."

"That is exactly it," replied Grandmother Terra. "The front channel of the arm on the Yin side is called Hand Tai Yin Lung. Now, looking at the two organs that are left, we have the Heart and the Pericardium. The Pericardium surrounds the Heart and is there to protect it. So, we will say that the Heart is deeper and less in contact with the exterior than the Pericardium."

"So the Pericardium is in the middle position and the Heart is in the back position. Is that correct?"

"Yes, that is correct," smiled Grandfather Terra. "So the three Yin channels of the arm are Front Tai Yin Lung, Middle Jue Yin Pericardium, and Back Shao Yin Heart.

"And now for the Yang side of the arm. As with the leg, we will use the Yin organs associated with the position to place the Yang organs. The first Yang organ we will place on a channel is the Large Intestine. We said that the Large Intestine is associated with the element metal, as is the Lung. The Lung was placed in the front Yin position. We will then place the Large Intestine in the front Yang position of the arm. So, the front channel on the arm is the Hand Yang Ming Large Intestine.

"The other Yang organ that we know is associated with an element is the Small Intestine. The Small Intestine is associated with the fire element, as is the Heart. The Heart is placed on the back channel on the Yin side of the arm. We then place the Small Intestine on the back channel on the Yang side of the arm. The back Yang channel of the arm is the Hand Tai Yang Small Intestine."

Sun nodded as they understood the information. They knew there was still a piece missing and asked, "You didn't talk about the middle position on the Yang side of the arm. What organ is associated with the Pericardium?"

"Very observant, Sun," responded Grandmother Terra. "There is still the last organ to be associated with the last channel. And this organ is somewhat of a mystery, as it doesn't have a clear equivalent in anatomy like all the other organs. This organ is called the Triple Warmer or Triple Energizer. In Chinese it is called the *San Jiao. San* means three in Chinese and *Jiao* can mean a place of energy, such as a burner. The use of three in this organ is showing that there are three areas where the organ can be found. There is the upper jiao or burner, which is from the clavicle to the diaphragm, there is the middle jiao or burner, which is from the diaphragm to the umbilicus, and the lower jiao or burner, which is below the umbilicus to the pelvic region. This is the organ that is associated with the Pericardium.

"So, the middle position on the Yang side of the arm is called the Hand Shao Yang Triple Warmer."

Sun could accept the new information, but wanted to make sure they got it. "Let me see if I understood. The last part of the name of the channel is associated with an organ. If the organ is a Yin organ, then it will be on the Yin side of the arm or leg, and if the organ is a Yang organ, then it will be on the Yang side of the arm or leg.

"The placement of the Yin organ and its function are how the organ is associated with a channel. If the Yin organ is below the diaphragm, then the Yin channel is placed on the leg, and if the associated Yin organ is above the diaphragm, the channel is placed on the arm.

"The function of the Yin organ in relation to the other Yin organs of the limb is used to decide which placement of the arm or leg the Yin organ will have. Yin organs with functions more in contact with the external world will be placed on a Yin channel that gets more sun. And Yin organs with more internal functions will be placed on a Yin channel that gets less sun.

"Once the Yin channels are placed on their channels, the associated Yang channel is placed next to them on the same position but on the Yang side.

"As there are only five elements, with each element having a Yin and Yang organ, and there are 12 channels, two extra organs are added on the arm.

"These two organs are the Pericardium for the Yin side and the Triple Warmer for the Yang side, and they occupy the middle position.

"The 12 channels and their positions are:

Front Foot Yang Ming Stomach

Front Foot Tai Yin Spleen

Front Hand Yang Ming Large Intestine

Front Hand Tai Yin Lung

Middle Foot Shao Yang Gall Bladder

Middle Foot Jue Yin Liver

Middle Hand Shao Yang Triple Warmer

Middle Hand Jue Yin Pericardium

Back Foot Tai Yang Bladder

Back Foot Shao Yin Kidney

Back Hand Tai Yang Small Intestine

Back Hand Shao Yin Heart."

"Perfect," exclaimed Grandfather Terra. "You got it all. We are utterly amazed at your capacity for this information."

Sun blushed and knew today's lesson was over.

17

EACH CHANNEL WILL HAVE ITS HOUR

The Channel Clock

Sun woke the next day with a sense of peace and yet also a sense of excitement for the day to come. They knew that they were almost at the end of the theory that they needed to understand the channels and would soon start really learning their physical form on the human body. It was 7 a.m. when Sun opened their eyes and was blinded by the rising sun coming in through the window. They felt warmed by the sun and also felt the movement in their body that directed them to the bathroom to evacuate the meal from yesterday, giving space to start a new day.

After taking care of their bodily needs they went downstairs to help their grandfather prepare breakfast.

Sun entered the kitchen to find Grandfather Terra already boiling some water and preparing some fruit. Without saying a word, Sun took the fruit from him and started to cut it. They were enjoying the moment of being next to their grandfather and just being. They noticed that they were happy in the moment and at peace. Now was not the time to ask and learn. It was not the time to think. That would come later in the day.

They spent the morning in silence. The only words spoken was when Grandmother Terra entered to say good morning. The rest of the morning was spent together enjoying the sounds that they didn't normally take the time to enjoy; sounds like the singing of the birds, the wind rustling in trees, the insects buzzing in the meadow. By the time they sat down to lunch they were all in almost a meditative state.

The sun had just reached the zenith of its arc and it was directly above the porch. No shadow was cast, as it was exactly midday. After a moment of enjoying the feeling of the high sun, Sun began to talk.

"I have noticed this morning that as the sun moved up to its highest point, we also changed our activities in relation to its position. It was a natural cycle that we were following, and I felt completely at ease with it. I know that the channels are in fact expressions of how the sun falls on the different parts of the body in relation to each other. And each channel has in its name the amount of sun it gets, if it is on the Yin or Yang side of the body, and an organ. In the classics you had me read there is also a passage about how each channel has a special time. Could you explain this concept to me?"

Grandmother Terra smiled. "Of course, we would be happy to explain the relationship of the channels to the cycle of the sun. This is called the Chinese biorhythm clock, or the Chinese channel clock. And even if it is lunchtime and not teatime, we will talk about it now. Well, after we eat, as thinking and eating at the same time are not the best of friends."

After a simple meal that was enjoyed by all, Grandfather Terra brought out some tea and poured each of them a cup. With her tea in her hand, Grandmother Terra started to explain.

"You did well to observe that the channels are expressions of the amount of sun each area of the body gets. And as the sun's shortest cycle is the passage of day to night, there is a relationship between the hours of the day and the channels. Remember that the flow of Qi in the body is a continuous flow that creates a continuous cycle. This cycle is determined by the sun. At certain times of the day and night different channels will have a higher concentration of Qi than at other times. It is important to remember that Qi is everywhere and always. When we talk about a channel having a particular time, we are saying that the Qi is more present in that channel at that time. There is always Qi in every channel at every moment, and the amount or concentration of Qi can vary throughout a day.

"Now let's use some logic. How many hours are there in a day?"

Sun responded without thinking. "Twenty-four hours, of course."

"And how many main channels are there?"

"Twelve main channels."

"So how many hours will each channel be associated with?"

"Well, 24 divided by 12 is 2. So, each channel will have a period of two hours when it has its highest concentration of Qi."

Grandfather Terra smiled. "Excellent, Sun. Each channel will have a period of two hours when it has its highest concentration of Qi. With that information established, let's move on to the next step. The cycle of day and night is determined by the amount of sunlight we get at any moment. Now if we think about the channels, we have two major types of channels, the Yang channels and the Yin channels. Which has more exposure to the sun?"

Sun laughed. "Obviously, the Yang channels do, as Yang is more related to the sun and Yin to the earth."

"Exactly," replied Grandfather Terra. "As the Yang channels are more related to the sun, we use the Yang channels to determine the times of all the channels on the Chinese clock. Now, how many Yang channels are there?"

"Well, there are three Yang channels of the hand and three of the foot. But there are only three names for Yang channels, so you could say there are three Yang channels or six. It depends on how you classify them."

"Brilliant. Let's use the channel names to classify them. We have three Yang channel names, Tai Yang, Yang Ming, and Shao Yang. Each name tells us how much sunlight the channel is exposed to."

Sun piped up, "Well not Yang Ming. You said it meant bright Yang. This doesn't tell us about the amount of sunlight but the quality of the sunlight. The other two tell us about the amount: Shao means lesser and Tai means greater. Am I missing something?"

Grandmother Terra responded, "Yes, you are correct, and with the clock we will see why it is called Yang Ming. So, we have three Yang channels and 24 hours. We will use the Yang channels to divide the day into different parts. If we divide 24 hours by 3, we get 8. So, we will separate the day into three different sections. The first section will be the morning, from 3 a.m. to 11 a.m., then the afternoon from 11 a.m. till 7 p.m., and finally the night from 7 p.m. to 3 a.m.

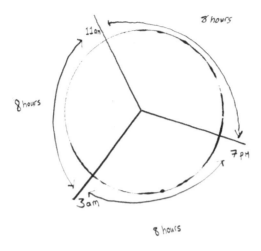

"Now, Sun, which time segment here gets the most amount of sun?"

"I would say the period from 11 a.m. to 7 p.m."

"Great. We will call this the *most sun* time period, and in Chinese that is Tai Yang. And the least amount of sun?"

"The nighttime—7 p.m. to 3 a.m."

"Correct again. So, this is called the *least sun* time, or Shao Yang. Now, the last time period, from 3 a.m. till 11 a.m. This period gets the *middle* amount of sun. And what happens during this time period? Especially in the middle of the time period between 5 a.m. and 9 a.m.?"

"Well, there is the sunrise then."

"And what does the sun look like at this time?"

"This morning it was blinding. It was very bright."

"So, we will call this period *bright sun*, or in Chinese, Yang Ming."

"So that is why the channel is called Yang Ming. It is referring to how we see the sun during that time. I get it."

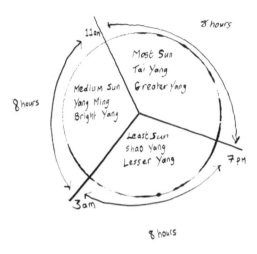

Grandfather Terra smiled at Sun's new understanding of Yang Ming. He continued where Grandmother Terra had left off. "We now have three sections of the day: the time with the most amount of sun, Tai Yang; the time with the least amount of sun, Shao Yang; and the time with the middle amount of sun, when the sun can blind us, Yang Ming. In each eight-hour segment we can now place some channels. We will place the Yang channels in the middle of their associated segment. So, the Tai Yang channel will be in the middle of the Tai Yang segment. The Tai Yang segment is from 11 a.m. to 7 p.m., and the middle four hours are from 1 p.m. to 5 p.m. The Shao Yang segment is from 7 p.m. to 3 a.m., and the middle of that segment is from 9 p.m. to 1 a.m. And the Yang Ming segment is from 3 a.m. to 11 a.m., with the middle being 5 a.m. to 9 a.m. These middle times are the times of the respective channels.

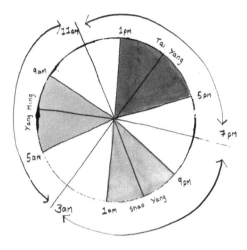

"Now, Sun, do you remember which way the Yang channels flow?"

"Yes, of course. The Yang channels are related more to the sun, so they start above and go down to the earth."

"Perfect. So, Yang starts above and moves down. Now, of the hands and the legs, which is more above?"

"The hands, silly. What kind of question is that?"

"Obviously a silly one. So, the Yang channels start in the hands and finish in the feet. Therefore, in the four-hour period we will put the Yang channel of the hand in the first two-hour spot and the Yang channel of the foot in the second two-hour spot. For example, from 1 p.m. to 3 p.m. we put in the hand channel of the Tai Yang, and from 3 p.m. to 5 p.m. we put in the foot channel of the Tai Yang. So 1 p.m. to 3 p.m. is the time of the Hand Tai Yang Small Intestine channel, and from 3 p.m. to 5 p.m. is the time of the Foot Tai Yang Bladder channel. Can you figure out the other ones?"

Sun thought for a few minutes before answering. "I will try. I am not sure I remember all the organs related to the channels though. In the nighttime the middle section is from

9 p.m. to 1 a.m. This gets the least amount of sunlight, so I will put it in the channel that gets the least amount of sunlight. This is Shao Yang, because Shao means lesser. The first section is from 9 p.m. to 11 p.m., and as Yang starts from the sun and comes down to earth, and the hand is closer to the sun than the foot, I will put the hand channel first. So 9 p.m. to 11 p.m. is the Hand Shao Yang channel. Which would mean that the second segment, from 11 p.m. to 1 a.m., is the Foot Shao Yang channel. However, I must admit that I don't remember the organs associated with the Shao Yang channels."

"That is perfectly normal, Sun," said Grandmother Terra quietly. "It's more difficult to remember the associated organs for the Yang channels, because the organ associations follow the logic of the Yin channels. The Hand Shao Yang is in the middle position on the arm and the organ that is associated with it is the Triple Warmer. The Triple Warmer is paired with the Pericardium on the Yin side. And for the foot it is the Gall Bladder. How about the last segment?"

"OK, I remember now. The Yang organ follows the placement of the associated Yin organ in the five elements. The last section is the Yang Ming section, which gets the medium amount of sunlight. The first two hours are from 5 a.m. to 7 a.m., and that would be the Hand Yang Ming. The following section, from 7 a.m. to 9 a.m., will be the Foot Yang Ming. Now let me see. The Hand Yang Ming is in the front of the Yang side of the arm because that gets the medium amount of sunlight on the Yang side. The front section of the Yin arm gets the most amount of sunlight for the Yin. The most amount of sunlight means the Yin organ with the strongest relationship with the exterior above the diaphragm, as it is in the arm. So, the Lungs would be the organ in the front of the arm on the Yin side. The Lungs are the metal element and the Large Intestine is also the metal element.

The Large Intestine will be with the Hand Yang Ming from 5 a.m. to 7 a.m. And this explains why I went to the toilet when I woke up this morning at 7 a.m."

"Very good. The channel clock with only the Yang channels would look like this."

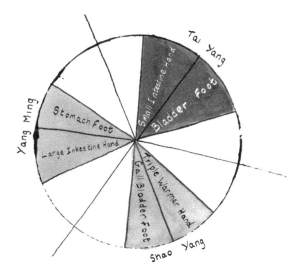

Sun looked at the image, nodding. Grandfather Terra was smiling, and continued, "Now, let us add the Yin channels. The Yin channels are placed next to the associated Yang channels using the five elements. So:

Before the Large Intestine goes the Lungs—metal

After the Stomach is the Spleen—earth

Before the Small Intestine is the Heart—fire

After the Bladder are the Kidneys—water

Before the Triple Warmer is the Pericardium—heaven (fire)

After the Gall Bladder is the Liver—wood.

"The full channel clock looks like this:

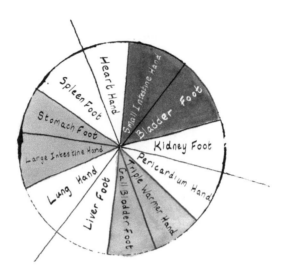

"Now let's add the times to it:

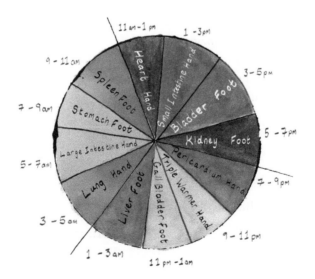

"And if we wanted to put all the information together it would look like this."

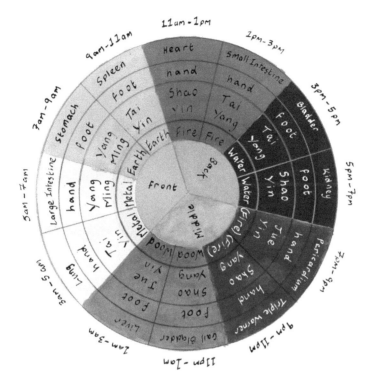

Sun looked at the full diagram and was enthralled. It was simple and made sense. They looked at their grandparents and said, "I understand the clock and the pattern. I would like to study this for a while before we talk more. I think there is a lot here for me to digest."

Both grandparents smiled and agreed. They had gone through a lot of information and it was time for a walk.

PART V

THE CHANNELS
ON THE BODY

18

CHANNELS IN THE ARM

Today was the day. Sun was excited. They had finally learnt enough theory to start learning the channels. They were impatient all day, doing the gardening and talking about everything except channels. Finally, it was teatime and they were ready. They sat down on the porch and took their tea. They were about to start talking when Grandfather Terra looked at them.

Grandfather Terra said, "OK, Sun. You have been patient and a good student. You have understood the theories of Yin and Yang, the five elements, Qi, the organs, the three divisions of the body, the flow of the channels, the Chinese names for the channels, and the channel clock. You are now ready to start seeing the channels on the body. Today we will talk about the arms. We will look at how the channels are positioned and their flow."

Sun was smiling and ready. "Great. I am excited."

Grandmother Terra started. "Let's put all the information we have gone over into use. We have already said there are three Yin channels in the arm and three Yang channels in the arm:

Hand Tai Yin

Hand Jue Yin

Hand Shao Yin

Hand Yang Ming

Hand Shao Yang

Hand Tai Yang.

"Each channel is associated with an organ and a position:

Hand Tai Yin—Lung—Front

Hand Jue Yin—Pericardium—Middle

Hand Shao Yin—Heart—Back

Hand Yang Ming—Large Intestine—Front

Hand Shao Yang—Triple Warmer—Middle

Hand Tai Yang—Small Intestine—Back.

"And the cross section of the arm would look like this:

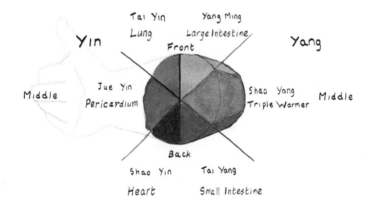

"We also saw the flow of the channels. The Yin channels start in the foot, go up to the thorax, and out to the hand. The Yang channels start in the hand, go up to the face, and then down to the feet. So, when we are looking at the arm, we will see that the Yin channels are going to be moving toward the fingers and the Yang channels are going to start in the fingers and go up to the shoulder.

"Let's see if you can now figure out where the channels are on the arm." Pointing to the palm side of her forearm in between the two tendons, Grandmother Terra looked at Sun and asked which channel it was.

Sun thought, trying to use all the information they had learned so far. "The palm side is the Yin side of the arm, so it is going to be a Yin channel. It is in the middle position of the arm, so it is a middle position channel. So, it is the middle Yin arm channel. The middle position on the Yin aspect of the arm gets the medium amount of sunlight. If I look at the table, I see that middle Yin on the arm is the Jue Yin, as Jue Yin gets the medium amount of sunlight. And the organ is the Pericardium. So, it is the Jue Yin Pericardium." Sun had a big smile and was clearly proud that they had put together all the information.

"Excellent," replied Grandfather Terra. "That is how the logic of all the theory can help us to understand which channel is where. Now, there are six channels on the arm; let's look at each one in relation to the others. Let's start with the Yin channels." Grandfather Terra took out a picture and showed it to Sun.

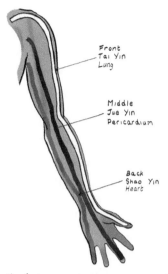

Yin (palmar aspect of arm and hand)
Goes from thorax to hand

"And if we look at the Yang side of the arm, we will see this."

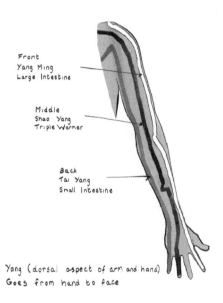

Yang (dorsal aspect of arm and hand)
Goes from hand to face

Sun looked at the two pictures and then at their grandparents. "It looks so simple. If I look at the fingers, they alternate from Yin to Yang.

Front:

Thumb—Tai Yin Lung

Index finger—Yang Ming Large Intestine

Middle:

Middle finger—Jue Yin Pericardium

Ring finger—Shao Yang San Jiao

Back:

Little finger (thumb side)—Shao Yin Heart

Little finger (non-thumb side)—Tai Yang Bladder.

"However, when I look closer there are areas where there are no channels. This doesn't make much sense."

"How perceptive you are," smiled Grandfather Terra. "Indeed, these are the channel lines that we use the most. They are in fact lines that connect the acupuncture points. The acupuncture points are specific points along the channels that can have targeted actions on the body. These are the channels that most people talk about. With that said, the channels are the whole segment. We use the pathways to line up all the acupuncture points that represent the same segment."

"I think I understand it. In the segments of front, back, and middle along the Yin or Yang sides there are places that have specific actions when used. The channel pathways are how these points line up. And also, the area around the points and in between the points will still be the same channel."

"That is it. Excellent," said Grandmother Terra warmly. "The arms are the easiest part of the body to identify the channels as there are no surprises. Next, we will look at the legs. In the legs there is one hiccup that we will have to understand for the legs to make sense. And that will be tomorrow's talk."

Sun knew that today's lesson was over.

19

CHANNELS IN THE LEG

After a night of dreaming about arms and channels, Sun woke to the sound of the birds chirping. They lay in bed a few minutes pondering the channels and feeling an inner joy at being closer to their goal of understanding the human body from a channel perspective. They delighted at how logical the system was and felt anticipation for another day of learning.

Sun went downstairs to have breakfast and saw a lot of gardening tools ready for the day. Grandfather Terra greeted them with a smile and a bowl of porridge. "This morning we will see the fruit of our labor over the summer. We will be harvesting some of the crops," he said.

Once Sun had finished breakfast, they went upstairs to change into their gardening clothes. They met their grandparents on the porch, and they went out into the garden together. It was a beautiful summer day and they worked hard picking and pulling the vegetables out of the ground. It was around midday when Grandmother Terra asked Sun to stop moving. Sun was in a crouching position, taking some of the potatoes out of the ground, and looked up at their grandparents. Grandmother Terra said, "Look at the position you are in. This is the position of the rice picker. Take a look at your lower legs. Do you see on the Yin side of the leg how the muscle is casting a shadow on the shin bone? Remember that position when we talk about the leg channels later today."

Sun looked at the position of their legs. They saw that when they were crouching down like this, their muscle was hanging over the shin bone and it was difficult to see the shin bone. They had no idea why they would need to remember this; however, they trusted their grandparents, who must have had a reason, so they took a mental picture of their legs.

After a long and fruitful day of working in the garden, all three of them were happy to have a moment to relax and drink their tea. With all three sitting in their chairs sipping their tea, Sun looked up at their grandparents and said, "So tell me about legs."

Grandfather Terra gave a bit of a chuckle. "Of course. It must have been difficult for you today wanting to know more and having to wait until now to ask. So, let's get into it. We will start with the same logic as the arms. There is a Yang side and a Yin side, as you already know. Do you remember how we divide the Yin and Yang on the leg?"

Sun thought for a second. "I think the leg was divided into interior and exterior when the feet are parallel and facing forward. Like this," they said, pointing to their legs.

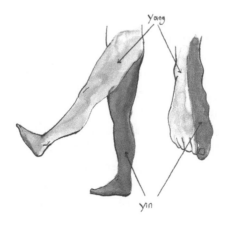

"That is correct," responded Grandmother Terra. "And now we will place the same three segments on the leg. We will have the front segment, the middle segment, and the back segment. And we will associate the channel names with the segments. We have Tai Yang, Yang Ming, and Shao Yang. The Tai Yang gets the most amount of sunlight, so is in the back position on the Yang side of the leg, the Yang Ming gets a medium amount of sunlight on the Yang side and will be on the front position of the leg, and the Shao Yang gets the least amount of sunlight and is on the middle position of the leg."

"Just like the arm," chimed in Sun. "And there are also the organ names associated with them, too. However, it is difficult to remember the exact order. I think it was Tai Yang Bladder, Yang Ming Stomach, and Shao Yang Gall Bladder, but I'm not sure."

"Perfect, Sun. You have a particularly good memory," said Grandfather Terra with a big smile. "Now, the Yang side of the leg follows the same logic as the arm and there are no surprises. But the Yin side has a slight complication. Do you remember the position we asked you to remember this morning? When you were squatting and picking the potatoes?"

"Yes. You told me to make a mental picture in my mind, and I am good at making mental pictures. I noticed that the muscle below the knee was casting a shadow on the front bone of the leg."

Grandmother Terra smiled. "Very good. And now let's see why we told you to notice that. We have the same three divisions of the leg on the Yin side—front, middle, and back. We also have the Chinese names that tell us how much sunlight that part of the body is getting. Tai Yin gets the most sunlight on the Yin side, Jue Yin gets medium sunlight on the Yin side, and Shao Yin gets the least amount of sunlight on the Yin side.

"When we were looking at the arm, we saw that the front

got the most amount of sunlight, the middle position got the middle amount of sunlight, and the back got the least amount of sunlight. Now, using the image that you have of squatting—which area below the knee got the most amount of sunlight?"

Sun thought for a moment. "The muscle part that was hanging off the bone got the most. Which I guess is the middle. But that's different from the arm."

"Exactly," said Grandfather Terra. "This is a particularity of the leg and the channels. Below the knee the middle part gets the most amount of sunlight, the front part gets the middle amount of sunlight, and the back part gets the least amount of sunlight. Above the knee the same order as the arms applies. So, above the knee the front will get the most amount of light, the middle the middle amount of light, and the back the least amount of light. Take a look at the following picture."

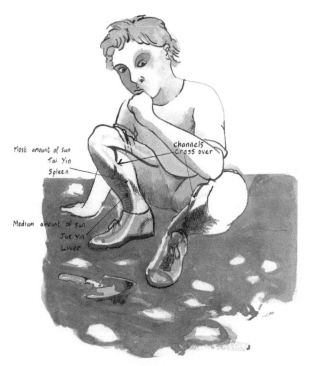

Sun said, "This is not really clear to me. Why would there be a difference of light above and below the knee?"

Grandmother Terra answered, "Good question. This is because of the way the muscles work in relation to the bones. When we walk or do any type of movement the body is balancing slightly forward. The fact that we are constantly slightly forward makes the relationship of the positions below the knee on the Yin side to the amount of sunlight different than the rest of the legs and the arms. So, we will see that the channels of the front and middle on the leg will cross at the knee. The Tai Yin, which gets the most amount of sunlight, will be in the middle below the knee and in the front above the knee. The Jue Yin, which gets the medium amount of sunlight, will be in the front below the knee and in the middle above the knee. The Shao Yang, which gets the least amount of sunlight, will be in the back Yin position all along the leg."

Grandfather Terra then asked Sun if they remembered the association of the organs to the channels on the Yin side.

Sun frowned. "I remember that the three Yin organs are the Liver, Spleen, and Kidney, but I don't remember which is associated with which."

Grandmother Terra smiled. "That is OK, Sun. There is a lot of information. We use the functions of the organs to associate them with the amount of sunlight. The more the function has contact with the exterior world, the more sunlight it gets. The Spleen is related to digestion, which is the exterior world, so it gets the most amount of sunlight—Tai Yin. The Kidney is the deepest organ in its functions and is associated with Shao Yin, and the Liver, which is in the middle, is associated with Jue Yin."

"Yes," replied Sun. "I remember that now."

Grandfather Terra took out a new diagram and showed it to Sun.

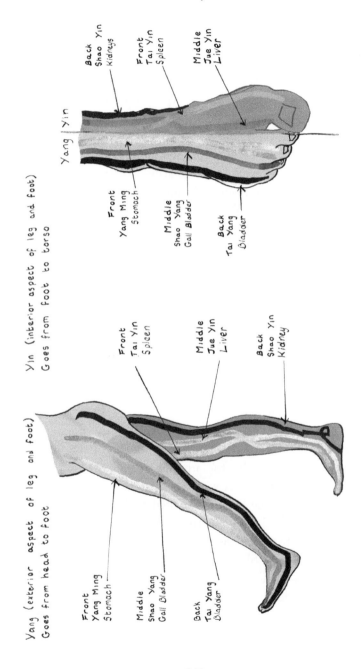

Yang (exterior aspect of leg and foot)
Goes from head to foot

Yin (interior aspect of leg and foot)
Goes from foot to torso

Front
Yang Ming
Stomach

Middle
Shao Yang
Gall Bladder

Back
Tai Yang
Bladder

Front
Tai Yin
Spleen

Middle
Jue Yin
Liver

Back
Shao Yin
Kidney

Yang Yin

Back
Shao Yin
Kidneys

Front
Tai Yin
Spleen

Middle
Jue Yin
Liver

Front
Yang Ming
Stomach

Middle
Shao Yang
Gall Bladder

Back
Tai Yang
Bladder

Sun looked at the diagram for a long time. They were taking it all in. They then started to make their commentary. "The first thing I noticed is that the foot is separated differently than the hand was. On the hand, the Yin side was on the palm and the Yang side was on the back of the hand. Here on the foot all the channels are on the top of the foot. The dividing line is the second toe. To the outside of the second toe are the Yang channels, and to the inside of the second toe are the Yin channels. Also, I don't see where the back Shao Yin Kidney starts."

"Very well observed," exclaimed Grandmother Terra. "The hands do in fact use a different dividing point between the Yin and Yang sides. This is because of the different structures of the hands and feet. And for the Shao Yin Kidney you are correct. The Kidney channel starts on the bottom of the foot. Remember that the Kidney is on the Shao Yin channel and Shao Yin means the least amount of sunlight. The bottom of the foot is the place where there is the least amount of sunlight, so this is where the channel starts."

"That makes sense," replied Sun. "Other than that, and of course that the Yin front and middle channels are different below the knee than above the knee, the leg channels are remarkably similar to the arm channels. I can see how this whole system is coming together. Grandfather Terra, can I have some more tea please?"

With a smile and a laugh Grandfather Terra served the tea, and the lesson on the leg channels had come to its conclusion.

20

CHANNELS IN THE TORSO

Sun woke up feeling the warmth of the sun gently caressing their face and body. They slowly got out of bed and went to look outside. They gazed out the window and saw their grandfather next to the pond doing some exercises. He was holding his arms out with his eyes closed, facing the rising sun. Sun thought he looked like he was absorbing the sun into his body, and they had the sense that their grandfather was communicating with the sun itself. Sun quickly got dressed and ran out to sit and watch their grandfather.

After a few moments, Grandfather Terra opened his eyes and smiled at Sun. "Come next to me, Sun, and stand in the same way as me." Sun ran next to their grandfather and tried to copy the posture and stance as best they could. Grandfather Terra came over and helped Sun by making some slight adjustments. They then stood next to each other absorbing the sun into their bodies. Sun had the desire to remove their top, and did so. They could feel the sun's rays penetrate deep and warm them.

After a few moments Grandfather Terra said, "Put your attention on your torso and feel where your body is accepting more light and where it is resisting."

Sun did as their grandfather suggested. They observed, "In my upper body I can feel that the sun penetrates deeper, yet it goes down to my belly to warm me."

"Very good, Sun. Now, can you notice where the separation is between where you feel the sun penetrating more and where it penetrates less?"

"Yes," said Sun. "It is just below the spot where my ribs come together in the front."

Grandfather Terra smiled. "Exactly. That is called the solar plexus, and it is one of the main energy points of the body. We will use it as a reference point later when we look at the channels on the torso. Now, for the moment, let's enjoy the sun and then go have breakfast."

Later that day, sitting on the porch and drinking tea, Sun and his grandparents started their discussion about channels on the torso. Grandmother Terra asked Sun, "How did you enjoy doing the Qi Gong with your grandfather this morning?"

Sun looked a little confused and asked, "Do you mean the exercises with the sun? Is that called Qi Gong?"

Grandmother Terra smiled. "Yes. That is one of the many exercises of Qi Gong. It is a practice of cultivating the Qi in the body. Your grandfather and I practice it every day."

"It was really nice. I felt like I had more energy after and yet was more relaxed at the same time."

Grandfather Terra was grinning, and said, "Then you were doing it well. That is the sensation you can get after a good Qi Gong session. So, as you felt the sun on the torso you also felt that different parts of the torso had different sensations. You felt that the upper part was more receptive to the sun and the lower part was more internal. This is because the upper part of the torso is more Yang in relation to the lower part of the torso. With this in mind we can start to see how the channels are placed on the torso.

"As the area above the torso is more Yang, this is where we

see the channels of the arms begin or pass through on their way to the head. This is also where the Yin channels of the legs come to join the Yin channels of the arm. And the Yang channels of the legs pass through here on their way down to the feet.

"However, below the diaphragm we only find channels of the leg, both Yin and Yang. So, when we look at the channels on the torso, we look at them in two sections. Above the diaphragm, where we have all the leg channels, the Yin arm channels, and some of the Yang leg channels, and below the diaphragm, where we only have leg channels."

"Oh, that makes sense. It's like when we associated the channels with the organs. If the Yin organ was above the diaphragm then the channel was on the arm, and if the Yin organ was below the diaphragm then the channel was in the leg," said Sun, beaming with pride.

"Exactly. So, to study the torso we will start with below the diaphragm and concentrate on how the leg channels are placed on the torso. The other thing that is important to understand when we are looking at the body and the head is that the relation of front, middle, and back are slightly different."

"Do you remember this diagram, Sun?" Grandmother Terra took out a drawing from a previous teatime.

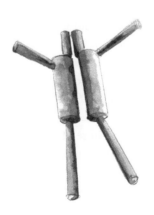

"Yes, I remember it. Each long round thing is a section. And the long round things are the same on the left and the right."

"Correct. The long round things, the cylinders, are the different sections of the body. When we saw the arms there were two cylinders for them, one for the left and one for the right. The same for the legs. And now we will see that it is the same for the body. The left side will be the same as the right side.

"Now, the question is, how do we determine the Yin and Yang separation and the front, middle, and back?" Grandfather Terra looked at Sun as he took a sip of tea. He could see Sun was trying to figure it out.

Finally, Sun gave up. "I don't see how we can use the same logic as we did for the arms and the legs. There was clearly a Yang side to the hands and arms that we could separate from the Yin side. It was the same in the legs. The only thing I could imagine here is that the front would be Yin and the back would be Yang. But that would create problems for the division of three for the front, middle, and back. Sorry, I do not see how we can use the same logic."

Grandmother Terra was smiling. "You see the problem, Sun, that is very good. The answer is we do not divide the torso into Yin and Yang and then the three divisions. We do it the other way around. We divide the body into the three sections first, and then within each section we have one segment that is Yin and the other is Yang. So first we divide each half of the torso into three vertical sections.

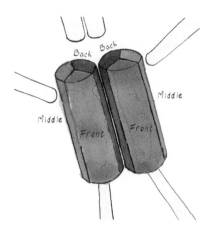

"We will then divide each section into two, one for the Yin and one for the Yang. Like this."

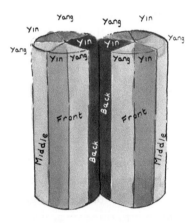

Sun looked at the pictures and contemplated them. "OK, so there are three main sections, front, middle, and back. And each section has two segments, one that is Yin and the other that is Yang. So, I would imagine that I would then take the placements that the channels are associated with in the leg and put those on the same placements on the tummy."

Grandfather Terra was smiling. "Nothing gets past you, Sun. That is exactly it. So, we said that the channels in the front are Tai Yin and Yang Ming; we will put the Tai Yin of the foot in the front Yin segment and the Yang Ming of the foot in the front Yang segment. We will do the same for the Shao Yin in the back Yin, the Tai Yang in the back Yang, the Jue Yin in the middle Yin, and the Shao Yang in the middle Yang. This is the general idea. Of course, we need to refine this idea a bit."

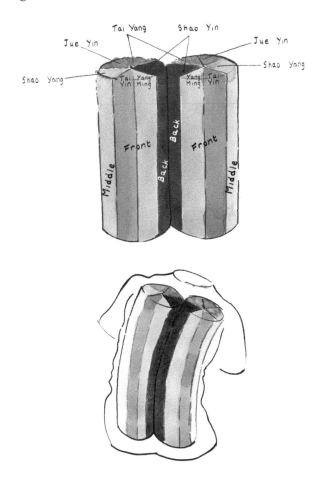

As Sun was looking at the images he noticed something. "The area of the back is also on the front of the abdomen close to the midline. How can a back channel be on the front of the body?"

"Well spotted, Sun," said Grandmother Terra. "Indeed, this is the case. The Foot Shao Yin Kidney channel is a back placement channel and yet we access it from the front, just next to the midline of the body. We need to access it from the front because it is deep inside the body, and in the back there is the spinal cord which we can't get through. So, it is drawn on the front of the body, but we treat it as a deep channel. Look at this picture:

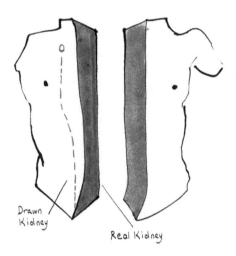

Drawn
Kidney

Real Kidney

"You can see that the real channel is deep in the back, and the accessed channel is on the surface in the front. It goes along the midline until it gets to the solar plexus, and there it moves out a little so the channel can be accessed in the areas between the ribs."

"Oh, that make some sense. OK. So, is there a pattern that helps to remember the channels in the torso below the diaphragm?"

Grandmother Terra responded, "In some ways, yes, and it is still a bit complicated. If we take the belly button and move away from it, we will see a pattern. Look at the following picture and say if you see it."

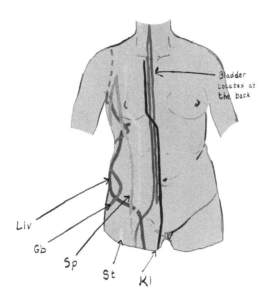

"The channels are Foot Shao Yin Kidney, Foot Yang Ming Stomach, Foot Tai Yin Spleen, Foot Shao Yang Gall Bladder, Foot Jue Yin Liver, and Foot Tai Yang Bladder. So I see that they alternate from Yin to Yang. There are the three sections: front, middle, and back."

"That is correct, Sun," Grandfather Terra chimed in. "That is the pattern—alternating from Yin to Yang. In the sections the middle channels cross over each other a few times. But other than that, you found the pattern. Now to be honest, it takes a little more work to remember the abdominal channels than the other areas of the body, but you have the basic principle. The last piece to add is the Yin channels of the arms. These are all in the upper chest and you can see them here:

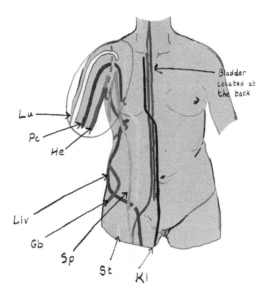

"If you go from the top to the bottom of the shoulder you get top (Hand Tai Yin Lung), middle (Hand Jue Yin Pericardium), and bottom (Hand Shao Yin Heart)."

Sun looked spent. "OK. This has definitely been the most complex lesson we've had so far. I think I need a good break."

Everyone laughed and drank their tea.

21

CHANNELS IN THE HEAD

Sun awoke the next morning with the sun gently warming their head as it entered the room through the window. They could feel the warmth caressing their cheek. As they got out of bed, they started to ponder on how the channels are placed on the head. They thought it must be similar to the torso but was not sure. Sun realized they were using these thoughts to distract them from the fact that they would be going back to their parents tomorrow. Their three weeks' holiday with their grandparents was almost over. Sun was excited to be seeing their parents and sad that they would miss their grandparents. They loved spending time with them and learning from them. The grandparents treated Sun like their equal and shared their knowledge and wisdom with them. It was more sharing than learning, and Sun never felt as much themselves as when they were in their presence.

At breakfast Sun told them as much. "You know, this is my favorite time of the year, spending time and learning from you both. I wish we could see each other more often. It's a shame you live so far away."

Their grandparents both smiled and just gave Sun a kiss on the cheek. That was all that needed to be said.

The day passed like all the others: having breakfast

together, working in the garden, going for a walk and having a picnic for lunch, resting after the afternoon walk, and then having tea on the front porch. Grandfather Terra said that repeating the normal routine on the last day would help reinforce the whole time they spent together, rather than doing something different which could confuse the memory. Start and finish with routine, surprise in the middle. Sort of like a sandwich—easier to hold and easier to eat, and still delicious.

Teatime was upon them. Grandfather Terra started pouring the tea while Grandmother Terra brought out the notebook. Once they were all sitting down, Grandmother Terra looked at Sun and said, "Well, as you can guess, today we are going to look at the last part of the body. The head. How do you think the channels will be placed here?"

Sun was ready for this question. They had been thinking about it all day. "I think it will be like the body in the divisions. There will be a left half and a right half. Each half will have three parts: front, middle, and back. But I could not figure out which would be where. Also, yesterday we looked at the torso. I noticed that the Yin channels of the foot ended in the torso and the Yin channels of the hand started in the torso. This would mean that there are no Yin channels in the head."

Grandfather Terra was smiling as always after hearing Sun explain something. A mix of pride and love were beaming from his eyes. "Very good, Sun. You got the gist of it. As you mentioned, all the channels in the head are the Yang channels. This is true for the main pathways. When you go further in understanding channels you will see that there are some internal pathways where some Yin channels come up to the head. But for our purposes we will say that only the Yang channels meet in the head. And you are also correct about the divisions. The head is divided into left and right. All the channels on the left will be the same as on the right. And finally, the segments. We will use front, middle, and back again, but they are different than on the body."

Grandfather Terra went over to the table, picked up a coconut, and looked at Sun. With a bit of a laugh he said, "This is your head." And then with a perfect strike on the table he broke the coconut into two perfect half spheres. "Now, each half has the same channels on it. One is the left side and one is the right side." He passed a half to Sun and asked, "Now, where would you say the front, middle, and back of the head are on this half?"

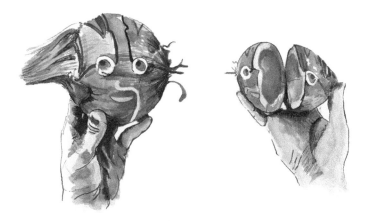

Sun responded, "The front is in the front, the middle in the middle, and the back in the back."

Everyone laughed. "Of course, Sun. That is true. OK, I will show you then. Let's take the acupuncture statue. We will hold the head like this:

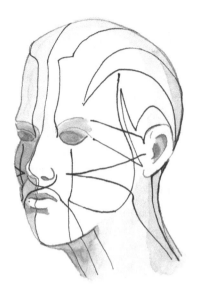

"We would put the areas like this:

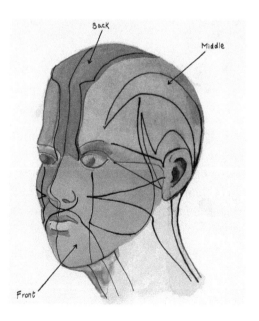

"The area below the eye, from the nose to the jaw line, would be the front; the area covering the ear and the side of the head to directly above the eye would be the middle; and the area above the eye closest to the midline going all the way to the back of the neck would be the back."

"OK, I see," piped up Sun. "When I was woken this morning by the sun on my cheek that was it on the front, my ear and side were the middle, and the center of my head was the back. Now, as we said before that the name of the Yang channels in the front are Yang Ming, and Yang Ming is related to the sunrise, this is why the first part of my face that touched the sun was the front."

"Yes!" exclaimed Grandmother Terra. "That is true. The front of the face gets the sun in the morning and is called Yang Ming, or Bright Yang, like the sunrise. So, you can see there are three general areas of the face. And in certain places they may overlap a bit. Now, the next thing to understand when we look at the head is the difference between the Yang channels of the foot and of the hand. To do this we will find a horizontal line to separate the head into above and below. Any idea which line we will choose?"

Sun responded, "When I was doing drawing class, they said that in the head the eyes are always the midline. So I would imagine that the eye line is where we would put the separation."

"Yes," said Grandmother Terra. "You see, school does teach you things too. Exactly, the eyes are the separating point. Areas above the eyes are associated with the feet channels, and areas below the eyes are associated with the hand channels. There are two exceptions to this, though. The front foot channel, the Foot Yang Ming Stomach, goes above and below the eye, and the middle hand channel, the Hand Shao Yang Triple Warmer, goes below and above the eyes. The reason for this is to allow for the flow of Qi."

Sun wanted to make sure they had got it. "So, the head is first broken in two like a coconut. Each half holds all the channels. The area below the eyes, the cheeks, the side of the nose, the mouth, and the jaw is the front. The area of the ear and the side of the head is the middle. And finally, the area above the eye closest to the midline and going all the way to the neck is the back. The foot channels are mainly above the eyes, except the Foot Yang Ming Stomach, which is in the front and goes above and below the eye. And finally, the hand channels are below the eye, except the Hand Shao Yang Triple Warmer, which is in the middle and goes below and above the eyes. Is that right, and can I have some more tea, please?"

Pouring some more tea for Sun, Grandfather Terra nodded. "You got it, Sun. Well done. There is one more thing we should look at before we see the channels on the head. Do you remember the flow of the channels? Where the Yang channels start in the hand and finish in the head and the foot Yang channels start in the head and finish in the feet?"

"Yes, I do remember that."

"Good. So we will now start by looking at the hand channels that finish in the head. Look at the following picture."

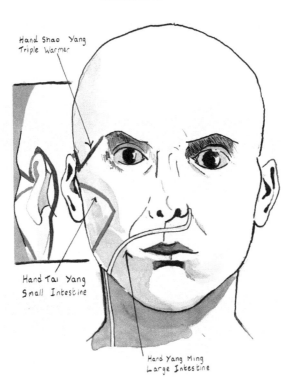

Hand Shao Yang
Triple Warmer

Hand Tai Yang
Small Intestine

Hand Yang Ming
Large Intestine

Sun looked at the picture while Grandmother Terra explained.

"The line on the front of the face is the front channel, so it is the Hand Yang Ming Large Intestine. You see that it comes up the side of the mouth, passes under the nose, and finishes on the other side of the nose. It is the only channel that crosses over the midline. And it does it under the nose. If you think about what comes out of the Large Intestine and how smelly it is, it is an easy way to remember that the channel goes under the nose.

"The line going around the ear is the middle channel, so it is the Hand Shao Yang Triple Warmer. It comes up the side of the neck, goes around the ear, and finishes at the end of the eyebrow. This is the only hand channel that goes above the eye.

"The line on the cheek is the back channel, so it is the Hand Tai Yang Small Intestine. This channel comes from the back of the neck and goes to the middle of the cheek and then to the ear. So, yes, this is a back channel, but it goes over the front area of the face. This is so it can connect to the foot channel in the back."

Sun looked up from the picture. "So, each hand Yang channel has a specialty. The front Yang Ming crosses over the midline, the middle Shao Yang finishes above the eye, and the back Tai Yang goes over the front aspect of the face."

"Well summed up," said Grandfather Terra. "And now we can add the foot channels."

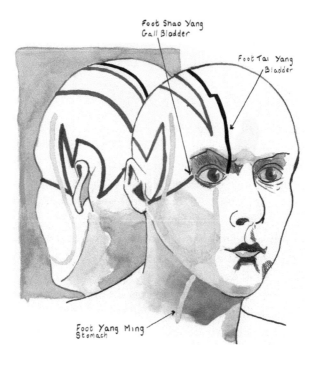

Sun took the new picture and looked at it while Grandfather Terra explained.

"The line on the cheek is the front channel, so it is the Foot Yang Ming Stomach. It starts just under the eye and goes down to the mouth, and then has two branches. The first goes along the jawline and goes all the way up to the top of the head. Another goes down from the corner of the mouth and over the front of the throat. This is the only foot Yang channel that goes below the eyes.

"The line that passes over the ear is the middle channel, so it is the Foot Shao Yang Gall Bladder. It starts on the outer corner of the eye and goes all over the side of the head, making many passes. It covers mainly the whole brain.

"The line running up from the eye is the back channel, so it is the Foot Tai Yang Bladder. It starts on the inner corner of the eye and goes up the forehead next to the center line. It passes over the top of the head just next to the center line and then down over the neck.

"When it comes to the foot channels in the head, the only exception is the front channel, which go over the face below the eye. The other two go over the hair and the forehead."

Sun nodded as they understood. "So to put it all together: All the channels in the head are Yang. The hand Yang channels come from the arm and neck to the face. Each of the Yang channels has a special quirk. Here they meet the foot Yang channels that go above the eyes and then down to the neck and body. The only foot channel that is special is the front channel, as it passes over the cheeks and jaw. The divisions of front, middle, and back are still used, but in a different way to the body, as the head is a sphere and the body is a tube."

"Perfect, Sun!" cried both grandparents together.

Sun smiled. "OK. I see it all now. The arms, legs, body, and head. I have one question that has come to mind. We separated the body and the head into the left and right sides, and all the channels were the same on the left or right side. What about the middle, between the left and right side? Are there any channels there?"

Sun's grandparents looked at each other and shook their heads. "Sun, you ask too many smart questions. We will answer that question over dessert, as it is now time to get ready for dinner."

"OK. Sounds good to me."

And they went to start preparing dinner.

22

THE MIDLINE CRISIS

The Governing and Conception Vessels

For their last dinner together before Sun was to go home the next day, they made a small feast. All of the vegetables they had worked on in the garden made a beautiful salad, and they prepared some meat that they slow roasted in the fire pit. The extra meat would be made into sandwiches for Sun to eat on the train ride home tomorrow.

After a wonderful dinner where they talked and joked about what a wonderful summer they had shared together, they prepared a fruit salad and Grandfather Terra made a wonderful cake with the cherries they had picked earlier that day.

Once they all had eaten the wonderful dessert, Sun asked their last big question again. "Are there any channels in the midline of the body and the head?"

While Grandfather Terra cleared away the plates, Grandmother Terra answered. "OK, Sun. Yes, there are two channels that go over the center of the body and head. These are two of what are called the eight extraordinary channels. The 12 channels we have looked at these weeks are the ordinary channels. They are ordinary because they follow the same patterns: they are all either Yin or Yang, start or finish in the hands or feet, occupy a position of front, middle, or back, are the same on the left and right sides of the body, and have acupuncture points on them.

"The eight extraordinary channels do not have all the same characteristics. We can separate these special channels into two groups: those that have only one channel in the body and have their own acupuncture points, and those that are on both sides of the body but use the acupuncture points of the ordinary channels.

"Your question is about the ones that have only one channel, and they are on the midline. The other six we will not worry about here."

Sun was nodding, and seemed to get it.

Grandfather Terra sat down, having finished clearing up. "These special channels we call vessels. This is because in Chinese they have a different word to describe them than the ordinary channels. We will talk about the Governing Vessel and the Conception Vessel. These are the two vessels that go over the midline, and they are quite easy to understand.

"As we have two vessels, what do you think will be the main definition of each vessel in relation to each other?"

Sun answered, "When we have seen two before, it was about Yin and Yang. So, I would imagine that one vessel will be Yin and the other Yang."

"Bright as usual, Sun," responded Grandmother Terra. "Now, we are talking about the midline. How would you divide the midline into Yin and Yang?"

"Well, there could be two ways: either above and below or back and front. As all the other channels have been on a vertical axis of the body I would imagine that the vessels do the same. So it would make more sense for them to be front and back."

"Very good. In fact, there is one extraordinary vessel that

does go horizontally in the body, but it is not either of these, so you are correct. One vessel will be in the back along the midline and one will be in the front. Which would be Yin, and which would be Yang?"

"As the back gets more sun than the front, the back would be Yang and the front would be Yin."

Grandfather Terra responded, "Perfect. So, the back-midline vessel is the Yang vessel and the front-midline vessel is the Yin vessel. One is called Du, and means *governing*, and one is called Ren, and means *conception*. Of these two actions, governing and conception, governing is more Yang and conception is more Yin. So, the Du Mai (Mai is the word for vessel) is the Governing Vessel and is in the back and Yang. The Ren Mai is the Conception Vessel and is in the front and called Yin."

Sun nodded. "OK, that makes sense. The back-middle line is Yang and the front is Yin. But there is one thing I'm not sure of. We said that the head was more Yang and that the Yang channels are there. If the front is Yin, would not the midline in the front of the face be Yin too? This doesn't seem to fit the logic of the rest."

"You are very perceptive," said Grandmother Terra, nodding her head. "Yes, you are correct. In the body the front of the body has the Conception Vessel, which is Yin, and the back, or the spine, has the Governing Vessel, which is Yang. The Governing Vessel goes up the neck, over the top of the head, down the front between the eyes, and finishes under the nose and above the lip, which is called the philtrum. The Conception Vessel goes over the front of the throat over the chin and to the tip of the tongue. So, the midline in the head and most of the face is Yang and part of the Governing Vessel.

"This is a good time to also tell you, Sun, that we have only been talking about the main pathways of the channels.

In advanced acupuncture books there are many more types of channels and internal pathways. All the other pathways help us understand why certain acupuncture points work or have other special functions. So, for example, the Conception Vessel under the mouth has two branches that go to the eyes. These branches do not have any acupuncture points on them, so they are not the main pathway."

Sun looked at his grandmother, confused.

Grandfather Terra chimed in. "We are telling you this so that when you see what we are giving you, you will understand it a little better."

As Grandfather Terra was saying this, Grandmother Terra took out a package. She handed it to Sun. Sun accepted the gift and carefully unwrapped it. Inside was a book. The book was hand drawn and had pictures of the channels.

"Thank you both so much." Sun got up and gave both their grandparents a big hug. They sat back down and started to look through the pages.

"This is our channel book. Each page will have some information about each channel and the trajectory. This is for you to look at and study. It can be a reference for you for all that we have learned this summer."

Grandfather Terra stood up. "Sun, we are enormously proud of you and have had a wonderful time this summer. And we now have to go to bed as tomorrow you have a big trip."

And with that they all went to bed for the night.

23

SUN GOES HOME

Sun woke in a state between excitement and sadness. Excitement to see their parents and friends, and sadness to leave their grandparents' home. They had had a great summer holiday. They had learned about Chinese philosophy, the human body, the five elements, the channels, and, most importantly, how much they appreciated and loved their grandparents. They thought it was a bit cheesy to think that, but they really felt it. When they were with their grandparents, Sun felt at ease and comfortable. And they loved that their grandparents took the time to share their knowledge and wisdom with them.

Sun went downstairs after finishing packing their bags and had a final breakfast with their grandparents. There was an unspoken feeling of accomplishment with all they had achieved this summer.

After breakfast was over, they got in the car and drove to the train station. They all waited patiently on the platform as the train rolled in. They made sure Sun had their lunch and all their bags. Sun's grandparents waved to them as the train pulled out. Sun felt tears running down their cheek and a feeling of warmth in their chest. The sadness was comforted by the love they felt from their grandparents, making it easier to bear.

Once out of sight, Sun pulled out the book their grandparents had given them. They saw that it was all handwritten and drawn by them. Sun flipped through the pages admiring their drawings, and a piece of paper fell out of the book. They picked it up and read it.

Dear Sun,

You are our favorite student. Thank you for letting us share our knowledge with you and for sharing yours with us. We are wiser for hearing your questions and explanations. This summer was a great collaboration and you are an amazing person. There is pride in our hearts when we think of you. We look forward to next summer with you.

Don't forget to look out the windows on the way home.

With all our love,
Grandfather and Grandmother Terra

Sun smiled and looked out of the window. This had been a great summer.

The Book of Channels

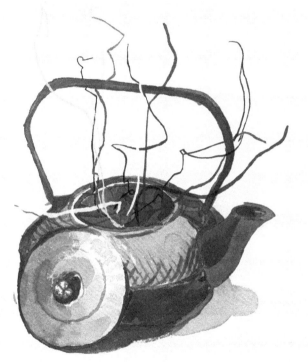

by the Grandparents Jerra

1. The Tai Yin Lung Channel

The organs of the Lung are situated above the diaphragm, so the Lung will be associated with a channel of the hand. Hand Yin channels start in the torso and finish in the hand. 'Tai Yin' means the most amount of sunlight on the Yin side of the body, which is in the front position.

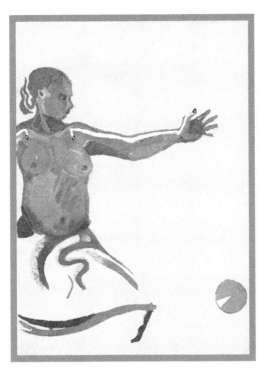

Hand Tai Yin Lung—Front position of the Yin side of the arm and hand

Organ	Lung
Arm or leg	Arm
Yin or Yang	Yin
Channel name	Tai Yin
Placement	Front
Starts	near the shoulder
Ends	Thumb
No. of acupuncture points	11
Element	Metal

2. The Yang Ming Large Intestine Channel

The Large Intestine is associated with the Lung organ, which is situated above the diaphragm, so it is a channel of the hand. Hand Yang channels start in the hand and finish in the head. 'Yang Ming' means a medium amount of sunlight on the Yang side of the body, which is in the front position.

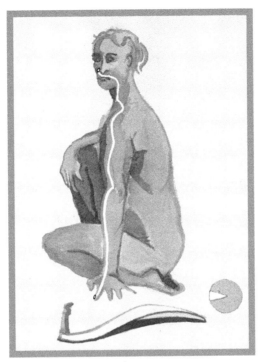

Hand Yang Ming Large Intestine—Front position of the Yang side of the arm and hand

Organ ———————————— Large Intestine
Arm or leg ———————— Arm
Yin or Yang ——————— Yang
Channel name ————— Yang Ming
Placement ———————— Front
Starts ———————————— Finger
Ends ———————————— Head
No. of acupuncture points — 20
Element ———————— Metal

3. The Yang Ming Stomach Channel

The Stomach is associated with the Spleen organ, which is situated below the diaphragm, so it is a channel of the foot. Foot Yang channels start in the head and finish in the feet. 'Yang Ming' means a medium amount of sunlight on the Yang side of the body, which is in the front position.

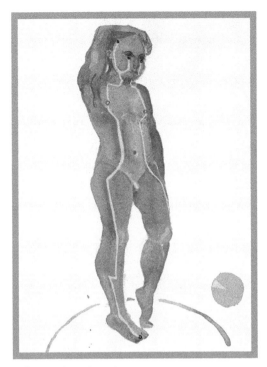

Foot Yang Ming Stomach — Front position of the Yang side of the foot and leg

Organ	Stomach
Arm or leg	Leg
Yin or Yang	Yang
Channel name	Yang Ming
Placement	Front
Starts	Under the eye
Ends	3rd toe
No. of acupuncture points	45
Element	Earth

4. The Tai Yin Spleen Channel

The organ of the Spleen is situated below the diaphragm, so the Spleen will be associated with a channel of the foot. Foot Yin channels start in the feet and finish in the torso. 'Tai Yin' means the most amount of sunlight on the Yin side of the body, which is in the front position.

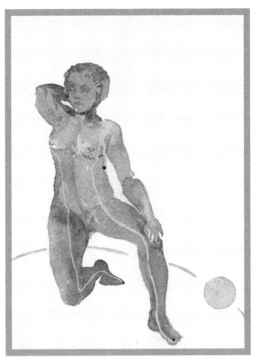

Foot Tai Yin Spleen — front position of the Yin side of the leg and foot

Organ ———————————— Spleen
Arm or leg ———————— Leg
Yin or Yang ————————— Yin
Channel name ———————— Tai Yin
Placement ———————— Front
Starts ———————————— Big toe
Ends ———————————— Thorax
No. of acupuncture points — 21
Element ————————— Earth

5. The Shao Yin Heart Channel

The organ of the Heart is situated above the diaphragm, so the Heart will be associated with a channel of the hand. Hand Yin channels start in the torso and finish in the hand. 'Shao Yin' means the least amount of sunlight on the Yin side of the body, which is in the back position.

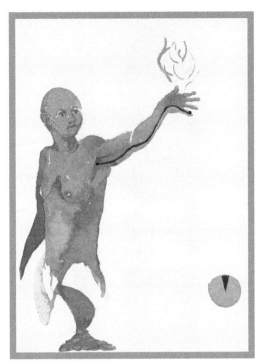

Hand Shao Yin Heart — Back position of the Yin side of the arm and hand

Organ ———————————— Heart
Arm or leg ———————— Arm
Yin or Yang ————————— Yin
Channel name ————————— Shao Yin
Placement ————————— Back
Starts ——————————— Armpit
Ends ————————————— Little finger
No. of acupuncture points — 9
Element ———————————— Fire

6. The Tai Yang Small Intestine Channel

The Small Intestine is associated with the Heart organ, which is situated above the diaphragm, so it is a channel of the hand. Hand Yang channels start in the hand and finish in the head. 'Tai Yang' means the most amount of sunlight on the Yang side of the body, which is in the back position.

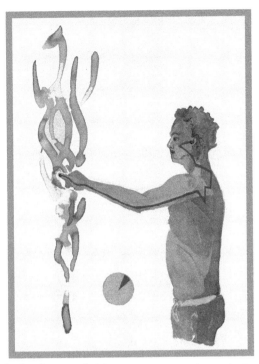

Hand Tai Yang Small Intestine—Back position of the Yang side of the arm and hand

Organ ———————————— Small Intestine
Arm or leg ——————————— Arm
Yin or Yang —————————— Yang
Channel name—————————— Tai Yang
Placement ———————————— Back
Starts —————————————— Little Finger
Ends ————————————————— Ear
No. of acupuncture points— 19
Element —————————————— Fire

7. The Tai Yang Bladder Channel

The Bladder is associated with the Kidney organ, which is situated below the diaphragm, so it is a channel of the foot. Foot Yang channels start in the head and finish in the feet. 'Tai Yang' means the most amount of sunlight on the Yang side of the body, which is in the back position.

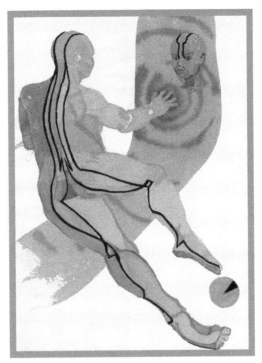

Foob Tai Yang Bladder—Back position of the Yang side of the foot and leg

Organ	Bladder
Arm or leg	Leg
Yin or Yang	Yang
Channel name	Tai Yang
Placement	Back
Starts	Eye
Ends	Little toe
No. of acupuncture points	67
Element	Water

8. The Shao Yin Kidney Channel

The organ of the Kidney is situated below the diaphragm, so the Kidney is associated with a channel of the foot. Foob Yin channels start in the feet and finish in the torso. 'Shao Yin' means the least amount of sunlight on the Yin side of the body, which is in the back position.

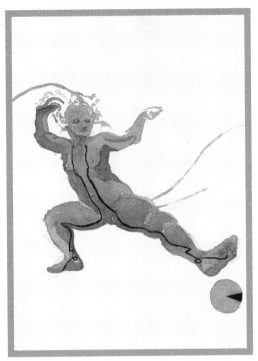

Foot Shao Yin Kidney—Back position of the Yin side of
the leg and foot

Organ	Kidney
Arm or leg	Leg
Yin or Yang	Yin
Channel name	Shao Yin
Placement	Back
Starts	Sole of foot
Ends	Collarbone
No. of acupuncture points	27
Element	Water

9. The Jue Yin Pericardium Channel

The organ of the Pericardium is situated above the diaphragm, so the Pericardium is associated with a channel of the hand. Hand Yin channels start in the torso and finish in the hand. 'Jue Yin' means a medium amount of sunlight on the Yin side of the body, which is in the medium position.

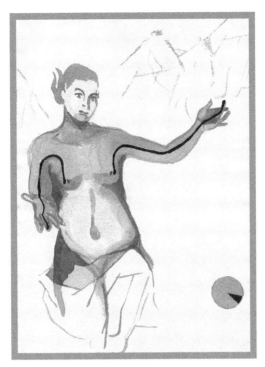

Hand Jue Yin Pericardium—Middle position of the Yin side of the arm and hand

Organ	Pericardium
Arm or leg	Arm
Yin or Yang	Yin
Channel name	Jue Yin
Placement	Middle
Starts	Next to nipple
Ends	Tip of middle finger
No. of acupuncture points	9
Element	Fire/Heaven

10. The Shao Yang Triple Warmer Channel

The Triple Warmer is associated with the Pericardium organ, which is situated above the diaphragm, so it is a channel of the hand. Hand Yang channels start in the hand and finish in the head. 'Shao Yang' means the least amount of sunlight on the Yang side of the body, which is in the middle position.

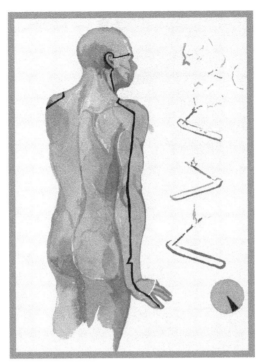

Hand Shao Yang Triple Warmer—Middle position of the Yang side of the arm and hand

Organ ———————————— Triple Warmer
Arm or leg ————————— Arm
Yin or Yang ———————— Yang
Channel name ————————— Shao Yang
Placement ————————— Middle
Starts ————————————— Ring finger
Ends ———————————— End of eyebrow
No. of acupuncture points — 23
Element ——————————— Fire/Heaven

11. The Shao Yang Gall Bladder Channel

The Gall Bladder is associated with the Liver organ, which is situated below the diaphragm, so it is a channel of the Foot. Foot Yang channels start in the head and finish in the feet. 'Shao Yang' means the least amount of sunlight on the Yang side of the body, which is in the middle position.

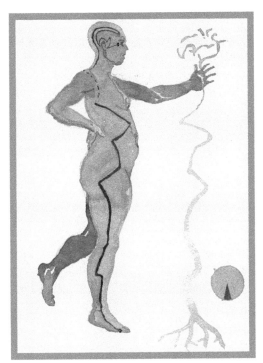

Foot Shao Yang Gall Bladder—Middle position of the Yang side of the foot and leg

Organ	Gall Bladder
Arm or leg	Leg
Yin or Yang	Yang
Channel name	Shao Yang
Placement	Middle
Starts	Next to eye
Ends	4th toe
No. of acupuncture points	44
Element	Wood

12. The Jue Yin Liver Channel

The organ of the Liver is situated below the diaphragm, so the Liver is associated with a channel of the foot. Foot Yin channels start in the feet and finish in the torso. 'Jue Yin' means a medium amount of sunlight on the Yin side of the body, which is in the middle position.

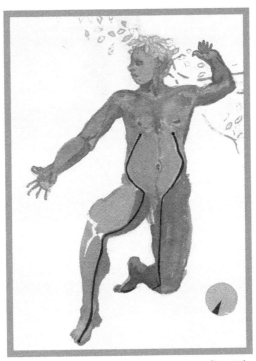

Foot Jue Yin Liver — Middle position of the Yin side of the leg and Foot

Organ	Liver
Arm or leg	Leg
Yin or Yang	Yin
Channel name	Jue Yin
Placement	Middle
Starts	Big toe
Ends	Rib cage
No. of acupuncture points	14
Element	Wood

13. The Governing Vessel

The Governing Vessel is associated with yang, so it runs along the back and the head. It starts at the lowest point of the spinal cord and finishes below the nose and above the mouth. As it is on the midline, there is only one channel.

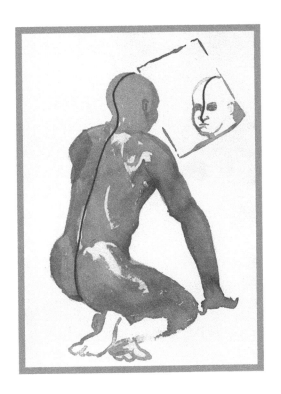

Organ ———————— None
Arm or leg ——————— None
Yin or Yang —————— Yang
Channel name————— Du Mai
Placement ———————— Back of body
Starts ————————— Just above anus
Ends ——————————— at the philtrum
No. of acupuncture points— 28
Element ————————— none

14. The Conception Vessel

The Conception Vessel is associated with Yin, so it runs along the front of the body. It starts at the lowest point beneath the genitals, and finishes below the mouth and above the chin. As it is on the midline, there is only one channel.

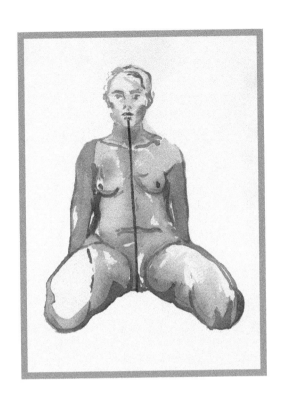

Organ ———————————— None
Arm or leg ——————— None
Yin or Yang ——————— Yin
Channel name———————— Ren Mai
Placement ——————————— Front of body
Starts ————————————— Between anus and genitals
Ends ——————————————— Between chin and lower lip
No. of acupuncture points— 24
Element ———————————— None